G000021958

PEMPHIGUS VULGARIS

AUTOIMMUNE BULLOUS DISEASE

DERMATOLOGY - LABORATORY AND CLINICAL RESEARCH

Additional books in this series can be found on Nova's website
under the Series tab.

Additional e-books in this series can be found on Nova's website
under the e-book tab.

DERMATOLOGY - LABORATORY AND CLINICAL RESEARCH

PEMPHIGUS VULGARIS

AUTOIMMUNE BULLOUS DISEASE

DANKA ŠVECOVÁ

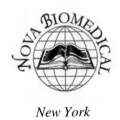

New York

Additional color graphics may be available in the e-book version of this book.

Library of Congress Cataloging-in-Publication Data

ISBN: 978-1-63463-317-8
Library of Congress Control Number: 2014959217

Published by Nova Science Publishers, Inc. † *New York*

CONTENTS

PREFACE

Pemphigus vulgaris remains in the forefront of dermatologic research. The knowledge of the pemphigus autoimmunity has basically changed. The first step in autoimmunity, the target antigens desmogleins (Dgs3 and Dsg1), which are the basis of the steric hindrance hypothesis and compensation hypothesis, have been largely reevaluated. New target autoantigens including acetylcholine receptors have the principal role in the "multi-hit hypothesis" which induces the signalling pathway that results in acantholysis. Elucidation of pathogenic steps allows investigating new therapeutic approaches which may meliorate prognosis of the diseases and improve morbidity and mortality.

This purpose of this book is to present the most recent scientific and clinically relevant information of pemphigus vulgaris. The knowledge of the pemphigus autoimmunity elucidates the background of the disease and shows the future of new approaches in its treatment. The most relevant problem of researching pemphigus is its rarity. Thus, the cooperation between multinational pemphigus centers should serve cohorts of patients for genetic, epidemiologic and clinical trials that could allow calculations and withdrawals.

Danka Švecová, MD, PhD
Professor of Dermatology,
Faculty of Medicine,
Comenius University,
Bratislava
Slovakia
danka.svecova@fmed.uniba.sk

SUMMARY

Pemphigus vulgaris (PV) is the most frequent condition inside the pemphigus group, especially in Europe and North America. It is the prototype of a genetically mediated disease. The HLA alleles associated with PV are well known. Recent studies found an association between disease severity and some HLA DRB1 and DQB1 alleles. PV autoimmunity with the prominent role of desmoglein (Dsg) 1 and Dsg3 autoantigens is discussed and gradually replaced with new autoantigens that are promoting "multiple-hit" hypothesis. The most discussed antigens to be the first target assaulted by PV autoantibodies are acetylcholine receptors. However, the Dsg1 and Dsg3 position is still important from a theoretical and clinical point of view because they possess the induction of autoantibodies that correlate with the clinical activity of the disease. The pathologic outcome of PV antibody-induced signalling is induction of the apoptotic and/or oncotic pathways resulting in apoptolysis. The final event is acantholysis restricted to the basal cell layer rending a "tombstone row" appearance. Recently, the influence of nicotine to PV has been evaluated. The interaction of nicotine with acetylcholine receptors on keratinocytes may help to increase cell-to-cell adherence. Despite PV having an unpredictable course, there are several studies that evaluated the association of certain clinical, epidemiological, immunological and genetic parameters that may influence the course and prognosis of the disease. The diagnosis of PV is derived from clinical and histopathological features, DIF, IIF or ELISA. Authorities recommended that is possible to discontinue immunosuppressive therapy in PV patients who have revealed a DIF negative result it they are at least 6 months in clinical remission. Most frequently, oral mucosa is the first appearance of PV. The mucosa on sites other than the oral cavity is considered to be more commonly affected than was initially recorded. Nose, ocular, laryngeal esophageal, genital and anal mucosa should be carefully examined using special assessment in cooperation with other specialists. Recently, new scoring systems have been introduced, as follows: the autoimmune bullous skin disorder intensity score (ABSIS) and the pemphigus disease area index (PDAI), which may help in evaluating severity and its development. Management of PV should be started with an evaluation of disease severity. The patient´s overall medical condition should be evaluated for whether there is a large risk of developing complications from immunosuppressive treatment. Corticosteroids are the mainstay therapy in PV, which is lifesaving but accompanied by multiple side and adverse effects. Adjuvant therapy is used to reduce the total dose of corticosteroids and to increase their immunosuppresion. Rapidly acting adjuvant therapies are used to control active disease. They include IVIG, plasmapheresis and immunoadsorption and rituximab. Slowly acting adjuvant therapies are used during maintenance and/or consolidation phases of treatment in order to reduce the dose of corticosteroids. The group of adjuvant therapies with slow onset of action includes azathioprine, cyclophosphamide, cyclosporine, methotrexate, mycophenolate mofetil and anti-inflammatory drugs (e.g., dapsone, antimalarials, gold, and tetracycline). Topical management disclosed new medications that promote healing, including topical immunomodulatory agents. Medications that promote healing in the oral cavity used until now in oncology may augment management in PV oral lesions.

Chapter 1

PATHOGENESIS OF PEMPHIGUS VULGARIS

ABSTRACT

Pemphigus vulgaris is the most frequent condition inside the pemphigus disease group, especially in Europe and North America. The incidence varies between 0.076 – 1.6 per 100,000 population, but is not known worldwide. Pemphigus vulgaris is the prototype of a genetically mediated disease. The HLA alleles associated with pemphigus vulgaris are well known and more than 95% of PV patients possess PV haplotypes. Recent studies found an association between the disease severity and some HLA DRB1 and DQB1 alleles. Pemphigus autoimmunity with the prominent role of Dsg1 and Dsg 3 autoantigens is discussed and is gradually replaced with new autoantigens that are multiple organ-specific and non-organ specific proteins, promoting a "multiple-hit" hypothesis. The most discussed antigens to be the first target assaulted by PV autoantibodies are acetylcholine receptors. However, the Dsg3 and Dsg1 position is still important from a theoretical and clinical point of view because they possess the induction of autoantibodies that correlate with the clinical activity of the disease. Autoimmunity in pemphigus vulgaris develops according to the rules of antibody mediated autoimmune diseases. Hitherto, the model of autoimmunity is investigated from the point of leading Dsg1 and Dsg3 autoantigens with the leading role of Dsg1- and Dsg3-reactive T cell in cooperation with B cells that line the anti-Dsg1 and anti-Dsg3 antibodies production. The role of Treg and Breg cells in the autoimmunity of pemphigus vulgaris remains to be determined, as well as the putative interplay between Treg and Th17 cells. The pathologic outcome of PV antibody-induced signalling is induction of the apoptotic and/or oncotic pathways resulting in apoptolysis. The final event is acantholysis restricted to the basal cell layer rending a "tombstone" appearance. Trigger factors that can induce pemphigus vulgaris in genetically susceptible individuals are considered to be the same as in other autoimmune diseases. Recently, the influence of nicotine to the pemphigus has been evaluated. The interaction of nicotine with acetylcholine receptors on keratinocytes may help to increase cell-to-cell adherence and to clear down acantholysis. Despite pemphigus vulgaris having an unpredictable course, there are several studies that evaluated the association of certain clinical, epidemiological, immunological and genetic parameters that may influence the course and prognosis of the disease.

INTRODUCTION

Autoimmune diseases, including autoimmune blistering diseases are acquired diseases with uncontrolled immune activity to own target autoantigens. Physiologically, this pathological activity is suppressed or it works as a regulation mechanism of unfavorable products removal thus these products do not induce damage to the tissue and cells containing target antigens. Autoaggressive reactions may develop as a result of immune homeostasis malfunction. Redundant autoantibody production or autoreactive T cells may damage self tissue with a serious defect on various organs or only on a specific organ containing target antigen. The disease is autoimmune in origin if the Witebsky postulates are established: the autoimmunity process is a reason of the disease; specific autoantibodies in human induced by target autoantigen may induce the same pathological process in experimental animal following immunization; the experimental disease passively can be transferred through the serum or T cells to experimental animal not previously immunized. [1]

Pemphigus vulgaris (PV) is a life-threatening mucocutaneous blistering disease that belong to the organ-specific autoimmune diseases mediated thorough autoantibodies directed to human epithelial target autoantigens. Autoantibodies are specifically directed to target desmosome components, i.e., desmosomal cadherins, namely desmogleins 3 (Dsg3) and 1that have a key role in keratinocyte cell-to-cell adhesion. The recent studies hypothesize that the first target antigens are acetylcholine receptors situated on the surface of epithelial cells, followed with other antigens of desmosomal or non-desmosomal origin. Autoreactive B cells produce autoantibodies to the target autoantigens upon regulation of autoreactive T cells. PV antibodies to various autoantigens are thought to inhibit the adhesive interaction of desmosomes leading to loss of cell-to-cell adhesion of keratinocytes by directs fashion as well as by signalling pathway. Passive transfer of PV antibodies to neonatal mice produces blisters that clinically, histologically and imunohistologically resemble those in patients with pemphigus vulgaris. Nevertheless, the etiopathogenesis of pemphigus vulgaris, particularly the role of genetic factors in the generation of autoantibodies that are relevant to disease development, remains poorly understood. As with all autoimmune disease, the etiology of pemphigus vulgaris is multifactorial, with complex interactions of genetic and environmental factors contributing to disease development and exacerbation.

Pemphigus vulgaris is a rare disease, for those affected it presents a lifetime physical, emotional, and monetary burden. New therapeutic modalities may improve prognosis and outcome of patients suffering from pemphigus vulgaris.

EPIDEMIOLOGY OF PEMPHIGUS VULGARIS

Autoimmune blistering disease pemphigus vulgaris is rare with an incidence of 0.076 – 1.6 per 100 000 population. The incidence of various forms of pemphigus, however, varies from country to country. [2, 3] There are six variants of pemphigus: pemphigus vulgaris, pemphigus vegetans, pemphigus foliaceus, pemphigus erythematosus, pemphigus paraneoplasticus, and drug-induced pemphigus. Hitherto, few large-scale epidemiological studies have been conducted on pemphigus. Pemphigus vulgaris is the most frequent and representative form of the pemphigus group, in both Europe and the USA, whereas pemphigus foliaceus is more prevalent in Africa and certain rural areas in underdeveloped countries, where it affects up to 3% of the population. [4] According to previous studies, pemphigus vulgaris accounts for 91.9% of all pemphigus. [5] The annual incidence of the disease has been calculated in various populations and differs among ethnic groups. The incidence of pemphigus vulgaris is higher in Jewish populations, in particular of Ashkenazi origin, in individuals of Mediterranean descent, in the Japanese and Indians as compared to the incidence observed in Western Europe or North America. [3, 6, 7] The incidence in Ashkenazi Jews was 2.7 per 100 000 population compared with 0.61 in the non-Ashkenazi population. [3] The mortality rate of Jewish patients suffering from pemphigus vulgaris is higher than that of non-Jewish patients, documented in a study by 26.2% of Jewish patients versus 3% of non-Jews. [8]

Several studies recorded divergent annual incidences among different ethnic groups living in certain territories, e.g., the overall annual incidence of pemphigus vulgaris in Macedonia was 0.51 per 100 000 population for ethnic Macedonians, which is in line with the incidence in neighboring countries. However, for the Romany the annual incidence was 2.4 and 0.1 for Albanians in Macedonia. [9] This is the only study about the epidemiology of the ethnic Romany population in European countries. It could be expected that this ethnic group could be included among populations with a higher incidence of pemphigus vulgaris. Annual incidence also differs in populations living in Germany. It is nine-fold higher in foreigners coming from southern European countries, namely Turkey and Italy, than in native Germans. [10] An internet-based patient survey study of pemphigus vulgaris collects wide-scale epidemiologic and demographic data relevant to the pathogenesis and clinical expression of pemphigus vulgaris in the USA. [11] The study is in accordance with the majority of other studies in literature that report a female predominance in pemphigus vulgaris (2.25), a predominant onset in the fifth decade of life (mean age of 51.8 years) and a predominance in the Ashkenazi Jewish population. A female preponderance has been observed in the majority of epidemiologic studies. The female to male ratio ranges from 1.1: 1 to 4:1 in various countries. The most frequent female preponderance is 1.2 to 1.5 seen in various European countries such as in France (1.2), Sicily (1.2), Bulgaria (1.11), Macedonia (1.3), Slovakia (1.6), the Mediterranean region of Turkey (1.4),and in Asian countries such as Korea (1.5), Northeast China (1.4), Iran (1.5), Israel (1.54), and India (1.16). [5, 9, 12-20] The female preponderance is still higher in several countries worldwide, reaching a level of 2 or higher, as in Switzerland (2.5), Croatia (2.0), and also in other countries such as Kuwait (2.0), Tunisia (3.2), and Japan (2.1). [21-25] It should be noted that there are only a limited number of studies on pemphigus vulgaris that do not show a female predominance. A higher frequency of pemphigus vulgaris in males than in females has been witnessed in Saudi Arabia (2.2), and Spain, in the territory of Seville (1.55), and in the territory of Malaga (1.22). [26-28] However, in Madrid the ratio recorded a female preponderance (1.08). [29] An equal sex ratio has been observed in pemphigus vulgaris patients from the Southeastern United States. [30].

Pemphigus vulgaris tends to appear in the fourth to sixth decade of life. The mean age at the onset of pemphigus vulgaris was registered in Israel as 53.5 years, Macedonia 52 years, Italy 54 years, Spain 57.4 years, and Switzerland 62.2 years. [9, 19, 20, 28, 31] The lower mean age of pemphigus vulgaris onset has been seen in multiple populations outside European countries, such as from Iran (42.2 years), USA (45.2 years), and Korea (44.3 years). [5, 11, 17] A higher mean age has been recorded in Germany, with 65 years in men and 51-65 years in women. [10] However, several studies recorded the gender difference at the onset age of the disease. In Greece, the difference was statistically significant. The mean age at onset of the disease was 55.8 years in females, while in males it was 59.6 years. [32] In Slovakia, the mean age of onset was also statistically different and lower than in the previous country, with 45.3 in females and 48.5 in males (27/44; 17/44). [33] In Spain, the onset timing was contrary to Greece. The mean age at the time of diagnosis was considerably lower in males than in females (50.1 vs. 66.3 years). [28] One of the discussed reasons for the difference in gender may result from the fact that estrogen exerts different influences on the development and function of the immune system in males and females, in which females may have a greater immune responsiveness to environmental insults, as well as to autoimmunity. [34]

However, autoimmune diseases are estimated to affect 4-5% of the population. [35] Generally, disorders of autoimmune pathogenesis may occur in individuals with a history of other autoimmune diseases. [36] Twenty percent of PV patients in an internet-based study from the USA also had been diagnosed with concomitant autoimmune disease, almost half of which concerned autoimmune thyroid disease. The second most frequent disease reported in family members was type 1diabetes mellitus. [11] The most frequent autoimmune disease in PV patients has also been documented, with thyroid autoimmune disease in 2.6% of pemphigus patients in Greece. [32] In the Slovak study, 22.7% (10/44) of PV patients suffered from an autoimmune disease other than pemphigus vulgaris, also accounting for the highest prevalence in thyroidal autoimmunity disorder (11.4%), followed by rheumatoid arthritis (4.5%), ulcerous colitis, psoriasis, and vitiligo (2.3% for each). [33] Another study revealed concomitant autoimmune diseases in 6.3% of patients with pemphigus vulgaris. Autoimmune thyroid disease was the most frequent (3.6%), followed by rheumatoid arthritis (2.7%). [37] Numerous studies documented autoimmune diseases in first-degree relatives of patients suffering from autoimmune conditions, including pemphigus vulgaris, reflecting that the genetic basis of these individuals is the most important background in susceptibility to develop the same or, more frequently, other autoimmune diseases. Pemphigus vulgaris does not occur in first-degree relatives, although 49% of those have been found to have low titers of PV antibodies. [37] These relatives are mostly the carriers of the genetic background of pemphigus vulgaris with a balance of good immune tolerance, which allows the induction of PV antibodies but does not allow a continuation of the autoimmune process to reach its goal, acantholysis. Even though, the literature review documented 25 families, comprising 53 patients, in which pemphigus vulgaris was diagnosed in more than one member. Relationships between those affected were mainly parent-child or sibling-sibling. [38] Recently, familial occurrence was also observed in another three families (two times in mother-daughter relationships and one in sibling-sibling). [39, 40] Moreover, one study documented pemphigus vulgaris in distant relatives in two families, one of Ashkenazi Jewish descent and the second of English-Scottish descent. [41] Taken together, these relatives shared a genetic background that predisposes them to develop a variety of autoimmune diseases, and in some valuable individuals it could also be pemphigus vulgaris. Another study evaluated the prevalence of autoimmune diseases in various degrees of relatives. There was a significantly higher prevalence of all autoimmune diseases in first-degree relatives (50.6%) of patients with pemphigus vulgaris compared with second-degree (34.3%) and third-degree relatives (15.1%). [42] However, these findings may be reflective of shared environmental or trigger factors relevant to the pathogenesis of autoimmunity. In the Slovak study, the first-degree relatives revealed autoimmune disease (11.4%), including diabetes mellitus (6.8%), rheumatoid arthritis and thyroidal autoimmunity disorder (2.3% for each). [15] Another study investigating the prevalence of autoimmune diseases in relatives found a statistically significant increase in the prevalence of insulin-dependent diabetes in relatives of pemphigus vulgaris patients and a significant increase in rheumatoid arthritis and a borderline significant increase in autoimmune thyroid disease. [43]

In addition to comorbid autoimmune conditions, a history of cancer was recorded in 11% of the PV patients in the internet-based patient survey of pemphigus vulgaris, which is higher than the reported prevalence of cancer in the general population of the United States (4.1% in 2007). [11] To date, no association has been established between neoplasmas and pemphigus vulgaris. However, there are numerous studies about an association of paraneoplastic pemphigus and lymphoproliferative neoplasm. Because the mean age at the onset of pemphigus vulgaris is in the fifth decade of life, the seemingly increased incidence of neoplasmas may simply reflect the fact that neoplasmas are more common later in life.

In conclusion, the epidemiological situation of pemphigus vulgaris is not known in all countries worldwide because of the disease's rarity. Despite this, the numerous studies documented that pemphigus vulgaris is the most frequent condition inside the pemphigus disease group, especially in Europe and North America. The highest incidence is documented in several populations, including the Jewish population, in particular of Ashkenazi origin, and in the Japanese and Indian populations. It seems that the Romany population may also belong to this entity. The age of onset of the disease is most frequently in the fourth to sixth decade of life, with a female preponderance. The prevalence of other autoimmune comorbidity is high in PV patients, mostly of thyroid autoimmune disease. Autoimmune comorbidity is also frequent in relatives; however, they do not suffer from pemphigus vulgaris.

GENETICS

Genetic and non-genetic environmental factors are believed to contribute to the dysregulation of normal immune tolerance, which ultimately leads to the development of autoimmune disorders, including blistering skin disorders. Autoimmune diseases, including pemphigus vulgaris, have a strong genetic component. Most of the literature on genetic susceptibility to autoimmune diseases has centered on the investigation of major histocompatibility complex (MHC) genes. MHC in humans is termed HLA (Human Leukocyte Antigen) and is located on chromosome 6p21. Increased frequencies of certain HLA alleles in patients with autoimmune diseases compared with those in healthy controls have been reported in various populations. Although specific class II alleles are associated with particular autoimmune diseases, a variety of confounding factors, including strong linkage disequilibrium between several HLA alleles, especially between DR and DQ, hinder the precise assignment of MHC susceptibility. HLA-associated susceptibility varies by ethnicity and may be further affected by other HLA- and non-HLA- associated genes, each further modified by variable penetrance patterns and strengths of association with disease development. [44]

The induction of immune and autoimmune actions is closely associated with HLA molecules, which perform a critical role in the presentation of an antigen to immunocompetent cells. HLA molecules class II create a groove that is competent to admit and bind foreign antigen fragments called immunogenic peptide containing 12 to 25 amino acid units. Immunogenic peptide overhangs from the groove on both sites. In the next step of immune response, the overhanging immunogenic peptide is presented to T cells. [1] HLA molecules perform a critical role in induction of the tolerance to self antigens. When the antigens defectively present themselves to immunocompetent cells or do not present themselves at all, this may induce the autoimmune process.

Pemphigus vulgaris is a genetically mediated disease. The genetic predisposition is associated with HLA genes. Generally, HLA DR alleles code competent molecules that are efficient at inducing the autoimmune process. Multiple HLA typing studies have been performed in pemphigus vulgaris in numerous worldwide populations. Early studies showed associations between pemphigus vulgaris and the HLA class II specificities DR4 and DR6. [45] More than 95% of PV patients possess one or both of these haplotypes. [46] Further molecular sequencing accentuated two HLA class subtypes, now known as DRB1 and DQB1. [47, 48] A variety of confounding factors, particularly the strong linkage disequilibrium within the HLA region (especially between DR and DQ), has made it difficult to precisely designate HLA risk alleles. [42] However, population studies of patients with pemphigus vulgaris have clearly documented that there are differences among the most prevalent alleles in various ethnic groups.

Each subsequent modified variable penetration may amplify the association with the disease. Positive associations with pemphigus vulgaris were found with the following HLA alleles: DRB1*04:02, *04:03, *04:06, *08:02, *08:04, *14:01, *14:04, *14:05, *14:08 in distinct population. [49-60] Two DQB1 alleles, DQB1*03:02 and DQB1*05:03 are associated with pemphigus vulgaris across the world, too. [49-53, 58, 61] At the DQA1 locus, DQA1*01:01, *01:04, *03:01 and *04:01 are associated with pemphigus vulgaris.

The currently mentioned allele names respect the new HLA nomenclature, which was officially introduced in April 2010. To address the ever increasing number of HLA alleles described, colons (:) were introduced into the allele names to act as delimiters of the separate fields. [62] The original designations (without colons) of the PV-associated alleles can be found in the quoted articles.

The association between HLA DRB1*04:02 with pemphigus vulgaris is particularly strong in the Ashkenazi Jewish population. [63] However, another eight alleles at the DRB1 locus were positively associated with pemphigus vulgaris in Caucasian patients with pemphigus vulgaris. HLA DRB1*04:02, DRB1*14:01, DRB1*14:04 were consistent with previously reported genotype analyses of French, Spanish, Italian, Sardinian, Argentinean, Iranian and Turkish populations. [52, 60, 64-67] A high occurrence of DRB1*14:01 was reported in Japanese and Mediterranean lineage, e.g., in French, Italian as well as in Brazilian and Argentinian PV populations. [50-53, 68, 69]

Recently, a new allele HLA DRB1*14:54 was discovered in association with pemphigus vulgaris, so far documented only in two studies. Allele HLA DRB1*14:54 was discovered only in 2005 and introduced to the HLA nomenclature in October 2005. [70, 71] In the meantime, this allele was included in DRB1*14:01 because they both differ in a single sole nucleotide. [70] Hitherto, several studies substantiated that DRB1*14:54 is probably a relative frequent of DRB1*14 allele. [70, 72, 73] Recently, DRB1*14:54 was detected in Caucasian European patients with pemphigus vulgaris living in the United Kingdom. [74] DRB1*14:54 allele was also discovered in PV patients in Slovakia and was not found in the Romany population who possessed DRB1*14:04. [75, 76] Interestingly, each Roma patient with pemphigus vulgaris (n=6) revealed haplotype DRB1*14:04-DQB1*05:03. In addition, HLA DRB1* 14:04 was increasingly reported in Chinese, Pakistani and French PV patients. [50, 57, 58] By reevaluating the PV population also from other destinations, the account of HLA DRB1*14:54 should be enhanced.

At the DQB1 locus, two alleles, HLA DQB1*05:03 and DQB1*03:02, are significantly elevated in Caucasian PV patients. [49] HLA DQB1*05:03 has been reported to be overrepresented in PV patients who are non-Ashkenazi Jews of Mediterranean descent. [51, 52, 56, 57, 64, 65] and in several other ethnic groups of other European [49, 57] and Asian countries, and others. [47, 53, 55, 57, 58, 61] However, the only significantly overrepresented allele at the DQB1 locus in Ashkenazi Jews in North America is DQB1*03:02. [50]

At the locus DQA1, three alleles are significantly elevated in Caucasian patients with pemphigus vulgaris, namely HLA DQA1*01:04, DQA1*03:01, DQA1*05:05. [49] In addition, HLA DQA1*01:04 was also documented in other PV patients, including Indian, Pakistani and European populations, namely Italian and French and in Caucasians in North America. [49, 50, 57. 61, 65] HLA DQA1*03:01 had an increased frequency in Japanese PV patients, Italian and Sardinian. [47, 65] Moreover, an elevated frequency of HLA DQA1*05:05 was described only in the North American Caucasian population. [49] In addition, HLA DQA1*05:05 and DAQA1*03:01 were also significantly elevated in Ashkenazi Jews in North America. However, HLA DQA1*05:05 is a novel association in Ashkenazi Jews in North America. [49]

Susceptibility to developing an autoimmune disease could also be influenced by the negative association of some specific alleles, which may play a protective role in the induction of autoimmune disease. Protective HLA class II genes may override the risk conferred by susceptibility alleles. Protective HLA alleles were documented in various autoimmune diseases, but no direct demonstration of their valid influence to downgrade risk of development of the disease has been confirmed. Protective alleles were documented in rheumatoid arthritis, type 1 diabetes mellitus, sclerosis multiplex, lupus nephritis and thyroid autoimmunity (Graves´disease). [77-81] The existence of protective alleles has been reported in multiple genetic studies of pemphigus vulgaris. Protective alleles in pemphigus vulgaris have significantly lower frequencies and display a negative association with pemphigus vulgaris, differing from population to population. The poll of protective alleles in various populations worldwide includes alleles DQB1*02, DQB1*06:01, DQA1*01:03, DQA1*05:01, DRB1*03, DRB1*13, DRB1*07, DRB1*11, DRB1*15. [47-50, 52, 53, 57, 61, 65, 64, 82] It is hypothesized that if an allele conferred a dominant protective effect, its frequency might be elevated in controls of those who were carriers of pemphigus vulgaris susceptibility allele versus noncarriers. However, no study to date has confirmed a direct preventive benefit of carrying a negatively associated allele. In the future, the measure of protective allele function in healthy relatives of PV patients, and correlating autoantibody titers with the presence of susceptibility alleles in combination with potentially protective alleles might elucidate the function of protective alleles. Three dimensional models of negatively associated MHC class II alleles allowing an examination of the pocket surface electrostatic potential conferred by the primary amino acid sequence may also yield an insight into how protective alleles could alter the presentation of self-peptides to ultimately thwart the activation of autoreactive T cells. [83]

The precise genetic studies evaluated three levels of analysis using linkage disequilibrium quantification, haplotype frequency and primary sequence polymorphisms, within the MHC class II pocket, with the determination of HLA DRB1*04:02 and DQB1*05:03 in Caucasian PV patients. It is estimated that more than 95% of patients with PV carry one of these risk allele. [42] The association between HLA DRB1* 04:02 and DQB1*05:02 is particularly strong in those of Ashkenazi Jewish descent. The high prevalence of HLA DRB1*04:02 among the general Ashkenazi population may account for the increased prevalence of pemphigus vulgaris in this ethnic group. [42] Only these two alleles, DRB1*04:02 and DQB1*05:03, possessed the required sequence polymorphism likely to confer disease susceptibility in pemphigus vulgaris. Analysis of the sequences and structure of these PV susceptibility alleles reveals key HLA peptide binding site pockets and residues that distinguish these molecules from non-disease-associated sequences. [49] Differences in the regulation of cytokines that induce the expression of MHC molecules or polymorphism in antigen-processing cytokines may also contribute to the existence of two modes of PV induction.

However, HLA class II associations with pemphigus vulgaris are well documented, and additional disease associations have been reported with several classic HLA class I molecules, including HLA A3, A10, and HLA B15, B35, B38, B44 and B 60. [48, 55, 84-86] The significance of these alleles in disease susceptibility remains unclear.

There are limited reports regarding non-classic HLA class 1b alleles, including HLA E, F and G and pemphigus vulgaris. Recently, an association between HLA E and pemphigus vulgaris was investigated. [87] HLA E mediates natural killer and CD8[+] T cell activity, suggesting a role in the regulation of autoimmunity. HLA E polymorphisms have been shown to play an integral role in various autoimmune diseases. [88] Although the precise mechanisms have not been fully elucidated, it is suspected that HLA E may be a key modulator in self and non-self discrimination and contribute to the development of autoimmunity. HLA E*0103X was significantly increased in PV patients. [87] It is suggested that HLA E*0103X has a potentially key role for HLA E in the control of ongoing autoimmune events in pemphigus vulgaris and the maintenance of peripheral tolerance.

The association of HLA G with pemphigus vulgaris was reported in Jewish PV patients. [89] Previously, it was reported that HLA G encodes proteins with structures similar to class I and II antigens using alternative splicing. [90] It is expected that HLA G may function not only as an antigen presenting protein, but also as an inhibitor of natural killer (NK) cells or cytotoxic CD8 T cells. [91] However, it is supposed that HLA G could be involved in a cascade of immune events leading to the production of anti-desmoglein antibodies. These mechanisms are currently being investigated. However, the exact mechanisms by which the HLA E and HLA G function in pemphigus vulgaris remain to be elucidated.

Non-HLA Genes

Although an association between pemphigus vulgaris and HLA class II alleles has been established, the genetic factors predisposing the disease are clearly polygenetic. Currently, there are non-HLA genes evaluated as having a definite link to disease. Hitherto, only a limited number of studies have been conducted to find suspected genes. Candidate for gene research responsible for autoimmune condition, including pemphigus vulgaris, are focused on possible autoimmune targets such as autoantigens, cytokines, lymphocyte structure or function related proteins, and general immune response molecules. One of the suspected candidates of the non-HLA gene is the autoantigen desmoglein 3 (Dsg3), which could possess polymorphism. A significant association between pemphigus vulgaris and the Dsg3*TCCTC haplotype was observed in British and northern Indian patients with pemphigus vulgaris. [92] Such a gene polymorphism could be possessed also in other autoantigens involved in the autoimmunity of pemphigus vulgaris as mentioned in the "multiple hit" hypothesis, especially acetylcholine receptors. The next study observed multiple immunoglobulin heavy chain polymorphisms and found an association with the VH gene VH3f-R4 of the immunoglobulin heavy chain constant region gene. [93] However, the kappa light chain constant region of immunoglobulins bears polymorphic markers involved in susceptibility to various autoimmune diseases, but did not possess polymorphism in PV patients. [94] Other possibilities in single nucleotide polymorphism (SNP) could possess transport associated antigen processing (TAP) genes in pemphigus vulgaris. [95] The study discoveries revealed conflicting results.

Numerous cytokine polymorphic variants are associated with the development of a broad spectrum of autoimmune diseases, including psoriasis vulgaris and systemic lupus erythematosus. [96, 97] Accordingly, the cytokine gene polymorphism may respond to the varying level of cytokine production involved in the autoimmune process. In a recent study, cytokine gene polymorphism of TNF-α IL-10 was discovered in pemphigus vulgaris. It was found that IL-10 ACC haplotype is associated with lower production of the cytokine and was significantly increased in PV patients. [98] An association with other low producer IL-10 haplotype (ATA haplotype) was confirmed in another report, thus providing further evidence for the possible role of IL-10 gene variants in genetic susceptibility to pemphigus vulgaris. [99] One of the IL-10 functions is to promote the production of immunoglobulins. On the other hand, it also exhibits immunosuppressive and regulatory effects. PV IL-10 may induce autoantibody production at the systemic level, whereas locally it could possibly downregulate the local inflammation, and suppress acantholytic process and prevent the blister formation. [100, 101] The association with low producer IL-10 haplotype may therefore contribute on a local level to the lower possibility to downregulate the local inflammation and subsequent acantholysis with blister formation. Other gene polymorphisms were documented in TNF-α, which is known as a strong pro-inflammatory cytokine whose increased level were detected in sera as well as *in situ* expression in lesional skin of PV patients. [102 -104] TNF-α in cooperation with other mediators may play a role in the induction of acantholysis in pemphigus vulgaris. [105] A high producer (-308 G/A haplotype) should be anticipated. Contrary to this premise, no quite significantly increased frequencies of low producer TNF-α were detected in PV patients (G allele; GG genotype and -308G/-238 G haplotype). [58] This result could be explained by the existence of linkage disequilibrium with HLA DRB1*03:01 allele, which was found to be present at lower frequency in PV patients enrolled to the study. [98] A similar result on the association of TNF-α single nucleotide polymorphisms with pemphigus vulgaris was also observed in other PV patients from the neighbouring population. [106]

Alteration in the protein tyrosine phosphatase N22 (PTPN22) has been shown to affect the threshold required for T cell activation and may be associated with several autoimmune diseases, including rheumatoid arthritis, type 1 diabetes and systemic lupus erythematosus. [98, 107, 109] However, the association between tyrosine phosphatase N22 alteration and pemphigus vulgaris in North American patients of either Ashkenazi Jewish or Caucasian decent was not established. [110]

A new field for investigation concerns the genome-wide association studies that have become the new approach for complex diseases. New strategies such as whole genome sequencing and DNA exon sequencing may discover novel variants and single nucleotide changes in the identification of disease susceptibility loci. The development of large-scale disease registries with correlated bio-repositories are needed to advance genetic studies in various studies, including pemphigus vulgaris. International cooperation is required to support the application of modern genetic technologies to this rare disease. It is likely that the combination of candidate gene and whole-genome approaches with newly considered study designs, including those involving integrated transcriptional and chromosomal profiling, will be needed to unravel the complex interplay of genes and the environment that drive the development of pemphigus vulgaris. [42]

Clinical Relevance of Specific Genetic Markers

The investigators try to focus on and define the links between specific genetic markers and clinical expression. The goal is to better understand the precise biologic and clinical consequences of carrying specific disease -risk and disease -modifying genes. Because the course of pemphigus vulgaris is frequently unpredictable, the identification of parameters that may predict the course and prognosis of the disease is desirable. Dhandha et al. documented that anti -Dsg3 antibody levels were significantly higher in patients carrying one or both of the disease-associated HLA alleles, namely DRB1*04:02 and DQB1*05:03, than in carriers of other HLA alleles. [111] Svecova et al. using an analysis of the HLA DR1* and DQB1* alleles with additional clinical parameters highlights the association of HLA DRB1*04:02 with severe pemphigus vulgaris and with the mucocutaneous type of pemphigus vulgaris. The frequency of these alleles was greater in patients with severe pemphigus vulgaris than in carriers of other HLA alleles. Moreover, the study documented an association of HLA DQB1*03:02 in patients with severe pemphigus vulgaris and in female patients. [15] These results were in concordance with their previous study, in which the authors documented more severe levels of the disease in female than in male PV patients. Simultaneously, they recorded a longer remission survival time in female PV patients compared with male PV patients. [33]

In the future, the goal of investigation is to find and exactly interpret genetic markers that may identify individuals at risk of pemphigus vulgaris using respectable genetic tests. This knowledge would help to predict the course of the disease and permit early intervention, as well as to predict the response to therapy and to order individual effective therapy. The research of pathophysiology should discover new therapeutic targets. These hotspots in the investigation of pemphigus vulgaris lead to a new era of personalized medicine.

AUTOANTIGENS IN PEMPHIGUS VULGARIS

The exclusive role of autoantigens desmogleins 1(Dsg1) and 3 (Dsg3) in pemphigus vulgaris pathogenesis which are the targets for autoantibodies in steric hindrance hypothesis, has been largely reevaluated. Nevertheless, new knowledge about multiple autoantigens and their equivalent antibodies has to elucidate the pathogenesis in new insight. Despite this, desmogleins (Dsg1 and Dsg3) are targets for antibodies that are probably developed as a sequence of the first hit and mostly reflect the severity of disease and correlate with flares and clinical exacerbation.

Desmosome

Desmosomes are specialized intercellular adhering junctions that serve to attach neighboring cells to each other. It is considered that these structures are destroyed in pemphigus autoimmunity through the interaction of autoantibodies to autoantigens. Until now, the primary autoantigens were considered to be desmogleins (Dsg), desmosomal cadherins, which belong to the core of desmosomes. Compensation theory tried to explain the localization of blister formation in pemphigus vulgaris and its various phenotypes, namely mucocutaneous and mucous phenotypes. Recently, the compensation theory has been undergoing review and a new theory of "multiple hits" is being discussed. The core of "multiple hits" hypothesis is acetylcholine receptors that play key roles in regulating keratinocyte adhesion and in maintaining their polygonal shape. Acetylcholine receptors are probably the first target to be assaulted by autoantibodies localized on the surface of keratinocytes. The other antigens, including desmogleins, could be involved in the autoimmunity process after this first step.

Desmosomes are situated in various tissues subject to intense mechanical stress, such as the stratified squamous epithelia of the skin, mucous membranes, as well as myocardium. Moreover, desmosomes are present in simple epithelia and non-epithelial cells, such as the meningeal cells of arachnoidea and the follicular dendritic cells of lymph follicles. Desmosomes are critical for tissue integrity, they are often remodeled and contribute to dynamic processes during development and wound healing. Furthermore, the desmosomal component may also play pivotal roles in keratinocyte differentiation, morphogenesis and tissue patterning, as well as in epithelial-mesenchymal transitions.

Desmosomes in the epidermis were first described by Italian pathologist Bizzozero in 1864. The term "desmosome" was established by Josef Schaffer in 1920 and has its origin in the Greek words for bond (desmo) and body (soma). [112] Originally, desmosomes were considered cytoplasm-filled intercellular bridges. However, using electron microscopy Keith Porter confirmed that desmosomes are contacts between adjacent cells, and he described desmosome ultrastructure in 1956. [112] The first detailed analysis of desmosome ultrastructure was performed by Odland in 1958. Currently, desmosomes are considered to be discrete plasma membrane organelles, to be one of a pair of interacting cells. Desmosomes in the human epidermis possess a diameter of about 0.2-0.5 μm, composed of two electron-dense plaques in each of the two cells that are separated by an intercellular cleft of 24-30 nm. [113] Desmosomal plaque appears to be approximately 40 nm in thickness and is associated with the inner leaflet of the plasma membrane in each cell. [114] (Figure 1.1 and Figure 1.2). Desmosomal plaque is composed of two dense structures with a less dense intervening region. Adjacent to the plasma membrane is the outer dense plaque (ODP), an extremely electron-dense structure that is approximately 20 nm thick. At the inner edge there is the inner dense plaque (IDP), which is less dense than the outer one and it's thickness is approximately 7 nm. The ODP exhibits transverse periodicity with an apparent distance of 2.6 nm, indicating that its structure is highly organized. Keratin intermediate filaments appear to make a looping attachment to the IDP. [114] The individual intracellular keratin intermediate filament cytoskeleton structures are connected in desmosomes, resulting in the formation of a strong and flexible frame as an intercellularly connected cytoskeleton throughout the epidermis. The schematic model of desmosome shows the relative position of the major desmosomal components (Figure 1.3).

Desmosome contains members of three protein families. Desmosomal cadherins form the intercellular adhesive interface, whereas armadillo and plakin family proteins build up the plaques. Desmogleins (Dsgs) and desmocollins (Dscs) undergo hemophilic and heterophilic binding via the interaction with the extracellular (EC) 1 domain of partner molecules on the same cells and on neighboring cells. The cytoplasmic domains are largely embedded in the outer dense plaque where they are associated with plakoglobin and plakophilin. In the inner dense plaque, desmoplakin links these adaptor molecules to the intermediate filament cytoskeleton and thus desmosomes link the keratin intermediate filament network to sites of strong intercellular adhesion. [115]

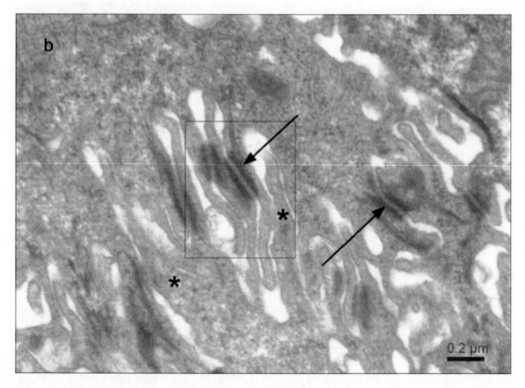

Figure 1.1. Ultrastructure of the desmosome. The electron micrograph of a keratinocyte of the stratum spinosum (*) shows the cytoplasmatic prominences of epidermal cells (b) which are close knitted through desmosomes (narrow). (Author)

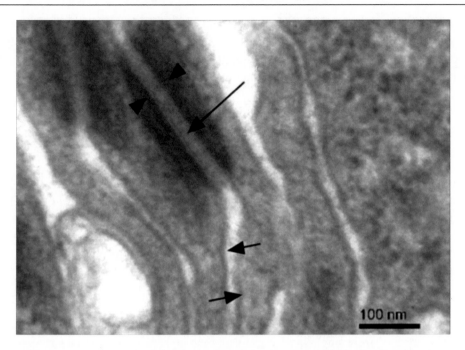

Figure 1.2. Detail of Figure 1.1. The electron micrograph of a desmosome shows discoid dense plaque (spike). The intercellular cleft of desmosome is filled with dense material (narrow). Short narrow shows plasmatic membrane of epidermal cells cytoplasmatic prominences. (Author)

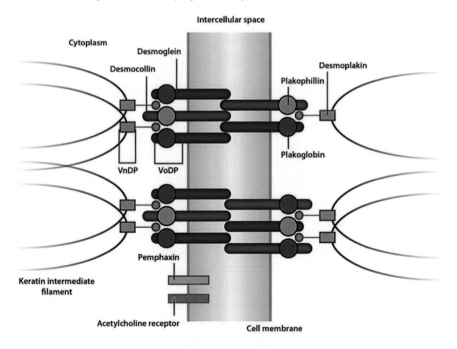

Figure 1.3. Schematic model of a desmosome showing the relative positions of the major desmosomal components in epidermis. The N-terminal halves of desmogleins (Dsgs) and desmocollins (Dscs) are bound to each other on the extracellular face of desmosomes (IDP, inner dense plaque), to form desmoglea, while their C-terminal halves bind to plakoglobin (PG), plakophillins (Pkps) and the N-terminus of desmoplakins (Dpks) to form the outer dense plaques (ODP). Modified from ref. [112]

In human epidermis, the cell-to-cell contact of epithelial cells is performed with two main forms of adhering junctions. The first junction is mediated by desmosomes, which serve as anchoring structures for keratin intermediate filaments to desmosomal cadherins, and the second junction is mediated by adherens junctions, which contain cell-type specific adhesion molecules from the cadherin super-family that are connected to actin cytoskeleton. Both differ in ultrastructure, biochemically, and functionally. In contrast with adherent junctions, which usually contain only one type of cadherin, desmosomes invariably contain two types of transmembrane cadherin molecules, desmogleins and desmocollins, as their adhesive glycoprotein components. The creation and maintenance of both intercellular connections, desmosomes and adhering junctions, constitute a dynamic process.

Desmosomes have historically been considered static junctions, but recent studies have uncovered multiple cellular functions of those cell differentiations, cytoskeletal architecture, cell migration and gene expression. The principal desmosomal molecular components are two desmosomal cadherins, desmoglein and desmocollin, two armadillo family proteins, plakophilin and plakoglobin; and the plakin family protein, and desmoplakin.

Desmosomal Cadherines

The desmosomal members of the cadherin superfamily, desmoglein (Dsg 1-4) and desmocollin (Dsc 1-3), are single -pass transmembrane glykoproteins that mediate cell-to-cell adhesion. [116] Both cadherines form the core of desmosome and their extracellular domains bind in a Ca^{2+}-dependent pattern, either in a hemophilic or a heterophilic fashion, to form a bridge between those components at desmosomes. Both show a tissue and cell-type-specific expression pattern. Some tissue, e.g., simple epithelia, expresses Dsg 2 and Dsc2 only. In stratified squamous epithelia, all desmogleins and desmocollin isoforms are present, although the expression of those is restricted to certain locations of the tissue. Dsg 4 was found to be the principal desmoglein expressed in hair follicles and could be a key mediator of keratinocyte cell adhesion in the hair follicle, and coordinates the transition from proliferation to differentiation. [117] Mouse models revealed genetic alteration of cadherines to cause severe damage to the fetus, including embryonic lethality (Dsg2, Dsc3), suprabasilar epidermal acantholysis and oral erosions (Dsg3). [118, 119]

The amino-terminal extracellular domain of both desmosomal cadherines possesses four cadherin repeats (EC1-4) and membrane proximal domain (EC5). [120] The EC1, EC2 and EC3 domains are located at the N-terminal region and EC4 and EC5 at the C-terminal region. The EC 1-4 domains are thought to be connected via flexible linkers to Ca^{2+}. The membrane-distal EC1 domain contains the adhesive interface necessary for trans-interaction. By establishing trans (juxtaposed) and cis (same cell) interacting adhesive complexes, desmosomal cadherines participate in providing mechanical strength to stratified epithelia. Desmosomal cadherines mediate both homo-and heterophilic binding. The cytoplasmic tail has an intracellular anchor (IA) and an intracellular cadherin-like sequence (ICS) domain. Desmogleins and desmocollins ICS domains provide binding sites for other desmosomal components such as plakoglobin. Additional domains found in the desmoglein cytoplasmic tail include the intracellular proline-rich linker (IPL) domain, a repeat unit domain (RUD) and glycine-rich desmoglein terminal domain (DTD). [121] The function of the desmoglein - specific cytoplasmic regions (i.e., IPL domain, RUD and DTD) is not known.

Desmocollins (Dsc1-3) are the second cadherin presented in the desmosome core. A recent study revealed that Dsc3 forms hemophilic binding and also heterophilic interaction with Dsg1, but not with Dsg3. [122] Desmocollins contain binding elements that allow the formation of interaction with desmoplakins, plakoglobin and plakophilins. [121]

Armadillo Proteins

Plakoglobin is the only essential desmosomal component that is also found in typical adherens junctions. [123] In epithelial cells, two major kinds of such plakoglobin-containing junctions are present, the adherens junctions anchoring actin microfilaments and the desmosomes anchoring intermediate filament bundles. In desmosomes, plakoglobin interacts with the cytoplasmatic portions of the cadherins (desmogleins or desmocollins) mediating Ca^{2+}-dependent cell-to-cell adhesion. It binds to the cytoplasmic sequence of desmogleins and desmocollins via its first three armadillo repeat domains. [124] Plakoglobin has been demonstrated to interact with other desmosomal plaque components such as desmoplakin, plakophilins and also with keratin intermediate filaments. [125] Mouse models revealed that inactivation of plakoglobin led to embryonic lethality due to the mechanical fragility of the myocardium and, when mice are viable, they involved subcorneal skin blisters and hair follicle dysfunction. Taken together, inactivation of plakoglobin showed a complex of phenotype that might involve both adhesion and signaling disorders. [126] It was documented that some mutants of plakoglobin bind distinctly to cadherines, including desmogleins. Ultrastructural analysis revealed that the desmosomes were greatly reduced in number and structurally altered, indicating that plakoglobin is essential for desmosomal stability. [127] There is evidence to suggest that plakoglobin may be somehow involved in regulating lateral association between other desmosomal components and desmosome size. Besides its function as a desmosomal stabilizer protein, plakoglobin is considered to be involved in nuclear signaling. It was documented that plakoglobin has weak transcriptional activity and cooperates with other transcription factors. [127] Plakoglobin is crucial to preserve epithelial homeostasis and is a key suppressor of the proto-oncogene c-Myc, which is required to stop proliferation and to allow terminal differentiation in keratinocytes. [128] Another potential target gene is the anti-apoptotic molecule Bcl-X_L, which might be repressed by plakoglobin. [129] Plakoglobin and desmoplakins are the only proteins expressed in all tissues, including skin epidermis, heart muscle, neuroepithelium and microvasculature, where intercellular junctions link to the cytoplasmic intermediate filaments network. [130] Plakoglobin is involved in binding with desmosomal cadherines as well as different classical cadherines such as E-, N-, VE- and M-cadherin. All these patterns indicate that plakoglobin contributes to plaque assembly and maintenance by interaction with cadherines occurring in the specific junctional structures. It is suggested that one of the architectural functions of plakoglobin is based on its ability to attach itself and other plakoglobin -binding molecules to cadherines, and thus to special sites of the plasma membrane. Plakoglobin is attracted and bound to different cadherines and different junctions with different kinetics. With *in vivo* models, truncation mutant of plakoglobin binds differently to desmogleins and classical cadherines. It is suggested that different sites of plakoglobin are involved in binding to the specific cadherines *in vivo* and that the availability of a specific binding segment may be regulated by changes of conformation or interaction with other proteins. [131]

The second member of armadillo proteins is plakophilin, which consists of three isomorphs plakophilin 1, 2 and 3. Plakophilins are found in the desmosomal plaque and in the nucleus. Plakophilins can directly interact with all other desmosomal components, including intermediate filaments via the amino-terminal half domain. Plakophilin 1 recruits desmosomal components to the cell membrane and induces desmosome assembly. [132] Mouse models revealed that genetic alteration of plakophilin 2 may cause embryonic lethality and heart defects. [133] Plakophilin 3 has been demonstrated to play an essential role in the maintenance of skin integrity. Plakophilin has been targeted in pemphigus vulgaris as demonstrated in the *in vitro* model. [134] Beside plakophilins' function in desmosome build up, they are considered to be involved in signaling mechanisms, both at cell borders and in the nucleus. [135] By these two activities, plakophilins may regulate cell adhesion and cell growth.

Plakins

Plakin family proteins are linkers between the cytoskeleton and cell-to-cell and cell-to-matrix contacts. The plakin family comprises desmoplakin, plectin, envoplakin and periplakin, which are found in desmosomes, but their function is less clear. Desmoplakin can interact with all other desmosomal proteins such as plakoglobin, plakophilin and desmocollin 1. [136] The linkage between the intermediate filaments and the desmosomal adhesion molecules is mediated by desmoplakin, plakoglobin and plakophilin. However, desmoplakin is considered to be the main linker protein between the desmosomal cadherin-plakoglobin complex and the intermediate filament cytoskeleton. [137]

Mouse models revealed that mutation in the gene encoding desmoplakin led to embryonic lethality, defect in the heart, skin and blood vessels, and neuroepithelium. The desmoplakin null embryos exhibited defects that have been appeared to be significantly more serious than those of plakoglobin mutant embryos. It is suggested that a participating cause of death might be a defect in vasculature, not reported for plakoglobin null embryos. [138]

The structure of desmosomes differs in various types of cells and tissues. The diversity of desmosomes has been reported in tissue differentiation and in the pathogenesis of several genetic diseases and some autoimmune responses against a specific desmosomal component which may affect only certain, but not all, desmosome-containing molecules. Some desmosomal components such as Dsg2, Dsc2, desmoplakin, plakoglobin and plakophilin 2 are ubiquitously expressed in all cells and tissues where the desmosomes are found. In epidermis, the plaque components such as plakoglobin, desmoplakin and plakophilin 3 are expressed in all cell layers. However, the skin and mucous membranes reveal inverse distribution in some of desmosome components, e.g., Dsg1, the major antigen of pemphigus foliaceus, is predominantly expressed in the upper epidermal layers, while Dsg3, the major antigen of pemphigus vulgaris, is expressed mostly in the lower epidermal layers. [120] However, an inverse expression pattern is also typical for plakophilins1 and 2, as well for desmocollin1 and 3. In contrast to Dsg1, which can be detected in some desmosomes on keratinocytes of the basilar cell layer, Dsc1 and Dsg 4 are absent in the basilar cell layer. [139] Dsg 3 and Dsc3 are present in oral mucosal epithelia, with minimal levels of Dsg 1. In addition, low levels of Dsg2 and Dsc2 are found in basilar cells of oral mucosa. [120]

Regulation of Desmosome Formation

Desmosomes in keratinocytes are the most important intercellular adhering junctions that provide structural strength for the epidermis. These junctions are connected directly with desmosomal cadherin proteins on the cell surface and anchor keratin intermediate filaments (KIFs) to their inner cytoplasmic surface to generate an intracellular KIF-skeletal scaffold through several associated proteins. The main role of desmosomes is to maintain epidermal adhesion and integrity. Despite these functions, desmosomes are structures that undergo regular remodeling. Recently, two cell-cell conditions are recognized, including stable hyperadhesion (Ca^{2+}-independent) and dynamic weak adhesion (Ca^{2+}-dependent) conditions. [140] Stable hyperadhesion is a unique feature of desmosomes that enables them to provide a strong link in the chain that makes up the desmosome-intermediate filament complex. The study of desmosome assembly in tissue culture showed that, when first formed, desmosomes could be disrupted by Ca^{2+} removal, but later became resistant. [141] These two different conditions are mutually reversible through cell signaling events involving protein kinase C (PKC) and epidermal growth factor receptor (EGFR). [140] Moreover, the difference in adhesiveness between Ca^{2}-dependent and Ca^{2}-independent desmosomes involves no quantitative change in the protein composition of desmosomes. [142] The majority of desmosome in normal epidermis are in stable hyperadhesion (Ca^{2+}-independent condition). Literature has documented that desmosomes of other tissue, including trachea, esophagus, tongue, liver and cardiac muscle are Ca^{2+}-independent, suggesting that this condition is the normal state for desmosomes in adult tissue *in vivo*. [143] Wounding of the epidermis is associated with dynamic weak adhesion (Ca^{2+}-dependent condition). This alteration in desmosomal adhesiveness is important for wound re-epithelialization. However, switching between the two adhesive conditions of desmosomes can be achieved by activation or inhibition of PKC, namely PKCα. It is suggested that specific phosphorylation by PKCα and perhaps other kinases, can modulate the structure of the desmosome plaque and is responsible for the conversation of stable hyperadhesion of desmosomes into a dynamic weak-adhesion Ca^{2+}-dependent condition and conversely, dephosphorylation is associated with stable hyperadhesion and phosphorylation with dynamic weak adhesion. [121] However, it is considered that adherent junctions play a very important role in desmosome regulation. Both β-catenin and plakoglobin situated in adherent junctions have been found as targets for EGFR -dependent phosphorylation. The EGFR activation and signaling is suggested to play an important role in cross-communication between adherens junctions and desmosomes. [144] In addition, adherens junctions are Ca^{2+}-dependent cell-cell junctions mediated by E-cadherin that forms intercellular bridges at their extracellular N-terminal. E-cadherin binds several associated proteins, among them plakoglobin situated at specific site of their intracellular C (carboxyl)-terminal domains, which, in turn, interacts with actin (microphilaments). [145] In a recent study, the elevation of Ca^{2+}concentration in keratinocytes culture induced the formation of adherens junctions in keratinocytes followed by binding of the desmosomes. It is suggested that adherens junction formation is a prerequisite for desmosome formation. [115] In addition, there could be a critical cross-talk present between adherens junctions and desmosomes for the regulation of cell-cell adhesion in keratinocytes.

Autoantigens on Keratinocytes

Both desmogleins (Dsg3 and Dsg1) participate in cell-cell adhesion at desmosomes. The pemphigus group can be divided into two major types resulting in the loss of keratinocytes cell-cell adhesion caused by acantholysis: pemphigus vulgaris exhibits autoantibodies to Dsg3 only, or to both Dsg1 and Dsg3, and pemphigus foliaceus to Dsg1. It is well established that pemphigus vulgaris is characterized by deep (suprabasilar) epidermal blistering; whereas pemphigus foliaceus exhibits superficial blistering that involves granular or superficial spinous cell layers. A distinct histopathology is followed by typical clinical signs, including blister formations on skin and mucous membranes in pemphigus vulgaris and only skin in pemphigus foliaceus. These differences between pemphigus vulgaris and pemphigus foliaceus are explained by compensation theory of Dsg1 and Dsg3. [146] According to compensation theory, in deep epidermis both Dsg1 and Dsg3 are present and Dsg3 compensates for the functional loss of Dsg1-specific autoantibodies, resulting in more superficial blistering in pemphigus foliaceus. In pemphigus vulgaris, where only Dsg3 autoantibodies are present, no epidermal blistering would occur because Dsg1 is considered to compensate for autoantibody-induced loss of Dsg3 binding (Figure 1.4 and Figure 1.5). However, acantholysis occurs in mucous membranes where Dsg3 is involved to be predominantly expressed desmoglein isoform, leading to the phenotype of mucosal -dominant pemphigus vulgaris. When autoantibodies against Dsg1 are also produced in pemphigus vulgaris, skin blistering occurs. In pemphigus foliaceus, mucous membranes are not involved; whereas in pemphigus vulgaris, mucosal disease is a regular finding, and skin involvement may additionally occur. These phenotypes usually correlate with different autoantibody profiles. Pemphigus vulgaris patients with only mucosal lesions reveal autoantibodies to Dsg3, but not to Dsg1. However, pemphigus foliaceus patients show autoantibodies to Dsg1, but not to Dsg3. Thus, in pemphigus vulgaris patients with both mucosal membrane and skin involvement we detect autoantibodies to both Dsg3 and Dsg1. [147] However, this model does not explain the absence of blisters throughout the epidermis in patients who have antibodies against both Dsg3 and Dsg1. According to compensation theory, oral lesions arise only in pemphigus vulgaris, because only those patients have the anti-Dsg3 antibody and only Dsg3 is present in the oral cavity. However, this theory does not explain why the lesions do not occur in all layers of the oral mucosa, since there is no Dsg1to compensate the inactivated Dsg3. Furthermore, this theory does not explain why both anti-Dsg3 and anti-Dsg1 antibodies, according to the theory, are required for lesions to appear on the skin in patients with pemphigus vulgaris, since the lesions arise only in the deep layers of the epidermis where there is any Dsg1 and where anti-Dsg1 antibodies should have no effect. [148]

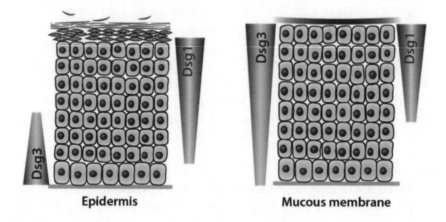

Epidermis   Mucous membrane

Figure 1.4. Diverse distributions of Dsg1 and Dsg3 in epidermis and mucosa. Modified from ref. [112]

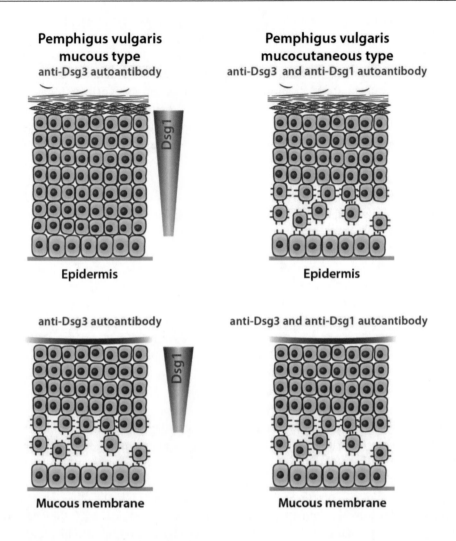

Figure 1.5. Compensation theory. Modified from ref. [112]

Compensation theory tries to explain the localization of split in both mucocutaneous and mucosal phenotypes of pemphigus vulgaris.

A multistep process is suggested in different mechanisms for pemphigus vulgaris and pemphigus foliaceus, resulting in different cleavage in epidermis. [149] Compensation theory marginalizes the complexity of homo- and heterophilic interactions of other known desmosomal cadherins, i.e., Dsg2 and Dsg4 and desmocollin 1-3. All these interactions are important to sustain the integrity of the epidermis. [150]

Recent studies confirmed that domain swapped molecules of the N-terminal EC1, EC2 and EC3 of Dsg1 and Dsg3 are Ca^{2+}-dependent. These epitopes are recognized by anti-Dsg1 and anti-Dsg3 autoantibodies, whereas recognition of epitopes on the EC4 and EC5 domains is Ca^{2+}-independent and not recognized. Thus, the major Dsg3 epitopes remained in the EC1 and EC2 domains. In the mucocutaneous type of pemphigus vulgaris, dominant epitopes of Dsg1 were present in the EC1 domain. In addition, paraneoplastic pemphigus (EC1 and EC4 domains of Dsg3) and pemphigus herpetiformis (EC1, EC2 and EC3 or EC4 domains of Dsg3 and EC1 domain of Dsg1, or EC2, EC3 and EC4 domains of and Dsg1) showed broader epitope distribution compared with pemphigus vulgaris. [151]

Epitope spreading is considered to be a phenomenon in which immune responses can spread over the disease course to recognize antigen epitopes that are different from the original target. Antigen specific autoimmune responses can spread to different epitopes on one protein (intramolecular epitope spreading) or to epitopes on other structural proteins (intermolecular epitope spreading). [152] In pemphigus vulgaris, intramolecular and intermolecular epitope spreading among extracellular domains on Dsg3 and Dsg1 is rare and has no correlation with the disease course. [151] Epitope transition is considered to be a rare phenomenon. Despite this, there are several case reports showing the shift between pemphigus vulgaris and pemphigus foliaceus. [153, 154] One possible explanation for this change may be epitope spreading. However, the disease progresses with augmented tissue injury caused by primary antibodies that results in the unmasking of neighboring proteins, to which secondary antibody responses are raised. The transformation of pemphigus vulgaris into pemphigus foliaceus may be a good example of the effects of epitope spreading. Accordingly, every target antigen generally contains several epitopes, each of which reacts with an antibody of different specificity and affinity. However, in the mucosal dominant type of pemphigus vulgaris the transition to a mucocutaneous type of pemphigus vulgaris may be managed by intramolecular epitope spreading from the EC5 domain to the EC1 domain of Dsg3, which is a critical step for following the intermolecular epitope shift from Dsg3 to Dsg1. [155]

The intramolecular epitope spreading raises an important role in the pathogenesis of endemic pemphigus foliaceus (Fogo Selvagem). In the preclinical stage, the EC5 domain of Dsg1 was reactive and then in the onset of the disease, the intramolecular epitope spreading activated EC1 and EC2 domains. The sera from Fogo Selvagem patients with active disease were reactive to EC1 and/or EC2 domains of Dsg1 and patients in remission showed reactivity restricted to the EC5 domain. [156] Moreover, intramolecular epitope spreading may also modulate remissions and relapses of Fogo Selvagem. On the other hand, the epitope shift did not occur in nonendemic pemphigus foliaceus. The EC1 and EC2 domains of Dsg1 immune reactivity prevailed across various activity stages, even upon remission. [157] The discrepancy may be due to the difference between endemic and nonendemic pemphigus foliaceus.

Various bacterial and viral antigens and pharmacological agents are the main exogenous causes of antibody responses that are directed to the structural proteins of desmosomal plaque. Fogo Selvagem is an example of molecular mimicry. The temporal and geographic clustering has led to the hypothesis of a triggering environmental antigen resulting in molecular mimicry with Dsg1, i.e., that autoantibodies directed to certain antigens of insect *Simulium* also react with desmosomal antigen Dsg1. [158] Medically induced molecular mimicry resulting in pemphigus vulgaris may be due to the formation of antibodies directed at sulfhydryl groups of certain medications, followed by binding to desmogleins. [152] Endogenous factors that result in molecular mimicry may include tumor antigens whose topology is identical or similar to that of desmosomal cadherines.

Other cadherines are considered as playing a role in the pathogenesis of blistering autoimmune diseases. The desmocollins (Dsc1-3) function is underestimated in cell-cell adhesion. However, a recent study demonstrated that Dsg3 cannot compensate for a loss of Dsc3 in the conditional $Dsc3^{null}$ mutant mouse that exhibit impaired cell-cell adhesion, leading to skin lesions resembling the blistering observed in patients with pemphigus vulgaris. [159] A recent study revealed that Dsc3 forms hemophilic and heterophilic interactions with Dsg1, but not with Dsg3. Loss of heterophilic Dsc3/Dsg1 binding may contribute to pemphigus skin blistering. [122]

By contrast, Dsc1 and Dsg3 seem to be the relevant target antigens in IgA pemphigus. In paraneoplastic pemphigus, the target antigens include Dsc1, Dsc2, Dsc3, BP-230, endoplakin, periplakin, plectin, Dsg 3 and other unknown proteins.

Some desmosomal proteins have not been described as possible antigens, as follows: pinin, desmiokin, desmokalmin and keratokalmin. The absence of antibody production against the latter group of desmosomal proteins is probably due to their intracellular localization.

The desmoglein compensation theory has clarified the basic pathophysiology of pemphigus; however, the theory cannot explain the process of blister formation satisfactorily. The "multiple hits" hypothesis indicated that besides Dsg1 and Dsg3, additional desmosomal and nondesmosomal proteins are present, which may serve as targets for autoantibody production. Both acetylcholine receptors, nicotinic and muscarinic, play key role in regulating keratinocyte adhesion and in maintaining their polygonal shape. [160, 161] It is believed that acetylcholine receptors could be the first target assaulted by autoantibody. Another keratinocyte surface antigen, pemphaxin, an annexin-like molecule binding acetylcholine, should be simultaneously targeted by autoantibody. [162] In addition, some mitochondrial proteins may also act as antigens. [163] Recently, over 50 human proteins have been reported to react with pemphigus autoantibodies. In addition to various desmosomal adhesion molecules and cell membrane receptors, immunologic and hematologic antigens, neuronal and oncologic antigens, and thyrogastric cluster antigens, were discovered to react with pemphigus autoantibodies. [150]

Taken together, these findings result in the conclusion that pemphigus autoimmunity is directed against multiple organ-specific and non-organ specific proteins, which promote a "multiple-hit" hypothesis. The most discussed antigens to be the first target assaulted by pemphigus autoantibodies are both acetylcholine receptors, nicotinic and muscarinic. Multiple adhesion molecules, as well as acetylcholine receptors and other keratinocyte proteins, have been referred to bind PV antibodies on the plasma membrane of keratinocytes and so initiate receptor mobilization, aggregation and downstream signaling as described in the "multiple hit" hypothesis. Desmoglein autoantigens Dsg3 and Dsg1 continue to be probably the only witness of autoimmunity in pemphigus vulgaris. However, their position remains important from a theoretical and clinical point of view because they possess the induction of autoantibodies that correlate with the clinical activity of the disease.

THE ROLE OF AUTOANTIBODIES

The basis of pathophysiology in pemphigus vulgaris is the separation of keratinocytes from one another by a process known as acantholysis. The primary event is associated with the presence of circulating autoantibodies reacting with autoantigens. These autobody-antigen bindings trigger keratinocyte detachment and deterioration of the cells. Besides autoantibodies, the mechanism of acantholysis involves various pathological factors, including cell-mediated cytotoxicity, proteolytic enzymes, pro-inflammatory and pro-apoptotic cytokines. The role of autoantibodies in pathophysiology of pemphigus vulgaris is well documented. The circulating PV antibodies are present in about 80% of patients with active disease and their titer usually correlates with disease activity. [111, 164-167] Furthermore, the tissue-fixed autoantibodies are present in about 80-95% of patients. [168] The presence of PV antibodies confirms the following events: newborns born to mothers with active diseases can develop transitory blistering as a result of transplacentar transfer of maternal autoantibodies and the injection of purified IgG from PV serum leads to blistering of the skin in newborn mice, with suprabasilar acantholysis in histology, corresponding to pemphigus vulgaris in humans. [169, 170] Transplacental transmission of autoantibodies from mother suffering from pemphigus vulgaris to her foetus is a "natural experiment" that results usually in the transfer of the disease to the neonates and strongly suggests that specific autoantibodies exert pathogenic effects. [169, 171] However, not always do the maternal autoantibodies that cross the placenta have to cause blistering diseases, in both pemphigus vulgaris and pemphigus foliaceus. [172] It appears that human placenta may modulate the expression of disease in neonate by operating as "a biologic immunoadsorbent" of pathogenic autoantibodies.

Although anti-Dsg1 and anti-Dsg3 antibodies, alone or in combination, are not exclusively responsible for triggering blisters in patients´ skin or mucosa, they have the diagnostic utility to differentiate pemphigus vulgaris from other blistering diseases. The value in patient management and prognosis, however, remains uncertain, and so anti-Dsg1and anti-Dsg3 antibody titers do not always correlate with PV disease activity nor do they predict exacerbation and relapse of the disease. [173, 174] Despite this, an analysis of autoantibodies profile revealed an association between anti-Dsg3 antibody levels and HLA DRB1*0402 and DQB1*0503. Patients carrying one or both diseases associated HLA alleles had significantly higher anti-Dsg3 antibody levels than carriers of other HLA alleles. [111]

It was originally thought that the clinical phenotype of pemphigus vulgaris is defined by the anti-Dsg antibody profile. Anti-Dsg1 antibody alone is associated with pemphigus foliaceus, anti-Dsg3 antibody alone with the mucosal phenotype of pemphigus vulgaris, and both anti-Dsg1 and anti-Dsg3 antibodies with mucocutaneous phenotype of pemphigus vulgaris. [147] Several studies reported a serological shift from $Dsg3^+/Dsg1^+$ to $Dsg3^-/Dsg1^+$ autoantibodies accompanied by clinical transition from pemphigus vulgaris to pemphigus foliaceus. [175] The transition from pemphigus foliaceus into pemphigus vulgaris has also been described; however, this progression appears to be extremely rare. [153] Despite the fact that anti-Dsg1antibody is considered to be a serologic marker of pemphigus foliaceus, up to 58% of pemphigus foliaceus patients and 43% of endemic pemphigus foliaceus (Fogo Selvagen) and in 20% of normal subjects living in an endemic area were documented to develop autoantibodies to both Dsg1 and Dsg3. [176, 177] However, anti-Dsg3 antibody revealed a low level and none of the subjects developed any obvious clinical phenotype of pemphigus vulgaris. Such a discrepancy between the antibody spectrum and clinical phenotype has also been found in pemphigus vulgaris. [175, 178, 179] In these studies, testing of anti-Dsg1 and anti-Dsg3 antibodies could not differentiate between various phenotypes of pemphigus vulgaris, i.e., 46% of PV patients did not have a mucosal or mucocutaneous phenotype predicted by their autoantibody profile. [179] In another study, 15% of PV patients with mucosal phenotype revealed both the anti-Dsg1 and anti-Dsg3 antibodies. [175] However, some studies documented the close correlation between anti-Dsg1 antibody titer and the course of skin lesions in patients with pemphigus vulgaris and pemphigus foliaceus, while the correlation between anti-Dsg3 antibody titer did not show correlation with the course of mucosal lesions, as well as with cutaneous involvement. [164, 171, 175] In some patients, anti-Dsg3 antibody can be absent at the time of diagnosis but subsequently could be developed. However, it can be present in complete remission and the absence of antigen exposition. [175] In addition, anti-Dsg1 or anti-Dsg3 antibodies have been detected in healthy individuals, relatives of patients with pemphigus vulgaris, and patients with irrelevant conditions. [180]

However, previous studies support the line of disease activity and anti-Dsg antibodies value, e.g., the correlation between clinical response and initial treatment in patients with pemphigus vulgaris and pemphigus foliaceus and the evolution of anti-Dsg1 and anti-Dsg3 antibodies titer, although the anti-Dsg1 antibody titer dropped more dramatically than the anti-Dsg3 antibody titer in patients who achieved complete remission. [173] However, this reasoning was not supported in all patients. During the long-term follow-up, a close relationship was documented between anti-Dsg1 antibody titer and the evolution of cutaneous lesions, especially in patients with pemphigus foliaceus, but not as markedly in patients with pemphigus vulgaris. [173] In remission, defined as no eruption for more than 3 months with minimal prednisone therapy, the anti-Dsg3 and anti-Dsg1 antibodies titer were detected in 46% of PV patients, in those who have had a high level of antibody during the active phase. [181] Patsatsi et al. compared the value of anti-Dsg antibody titer and disease severity measured by PDAI and ABSIS score. The anti-Dsg1 antibody titer correlated with the disease extent in cutaneous or mucocutaneous phenotypes, but the anti -Dsg 3 antibody titer did not correlate with disease severity. [182] A controversial report documented initially a low level of anti-Dsg1antibody, which increased during treatment and the anti-Dsg3 antibody titer remained at normal level during disease exacerbation. [183] This finding may keep the notion that anti-Dsg antibodies may "witness" rather than trigger pemphigus vulgaris, i.e., that the production of anti-Dsg antibodies is the result rather than the cause in pemphigus vulgaris. [184]

PV autoantibodies belong to all IgG subclasses as follows: IgG_1, IgG_2, IgG_3 and IgG_4. It is generally supposed that the pathogenic antibodies in the active phase of pemphigus vulgaris were the IgG_4 subclass, while in remission most circulating antibodies are IgG_1. [185, 186] It is thought that IgG_4 antibodies are pathogenic because they can recognize a different epitope to that of nonpathogenic IgG_1 antibodies. [185] Alternatively, IgG_4 may have an as yet unknown effector function that is not present in IgG_1, or a higher binding affinity for desmogleins. Warren et al. documented that the progression from a preclinical to a clinical phase of the disease, and also the transmission from remission into active disease, was associated with a subclass switching from IgG_1 to IgG_4 in pemphigus foliaceus. [187] The subclass of IgG_4 was associated with active pemphigus vulgaris and IgG_1 with remission of disease. [186, 188] However, some studies confirmed that both IgG_4 and IgG_1 are the predominant IgG subtypes found in PV patients in the active phase of the disease, while in remission IgG_4 levels remain higher than IgG_1 levels. [111] The same predominance was also found in pemphigus foliaceus. [189] However, about 50% of healthy unaffected relatives of patients with pemphigus vulgaris have circulating PV antibodies, with their subclass mostly belonging to IgG_1. [190]

It is unknown why many patients in remission continue to have clearly detectable IgG_4 in the absence of any clinical symptoms. One possibility of this event could be that anti-Dsg3 and anti-Dsg1antibodies remain in circulation during remission and are non-pathogenic rather than pathogenic. [185] Other antibodies such as IgG_2 and IgG_3 were detected in PV patients, but their role remains unclear. [189, 191] Another study discovered in PV patients with clinical remission a predominance of IgG_2 (75%) and IgG_4 (37.5%) subclasses. In their healthy relatives, circulating IgG_2 and IgG_4 subclasses were also detected in 60% and 23%, respectively. [192] In addition to anti-Dsg3 and anti-Dsg1-IgG antibodies, also IgA antibody was concurrently documented, which follows the antigen specificity of IgG. [193] Another study revealed IgE antibodies in a strong correlation with IgG_4 in the acute onset of the disease, but not in the chronic active phase or remission. In addition, IgE deposits were detected in the epidermis of acute onset pemphigus vulgaris. [194] Their relevance remained unknown.

It was previously established that most PV antibodies are directed against the extracellular domain of Dsg1 or Dsg3, and those antibodies are proven to play a pathogenic role in blister formation. However, the reactivity of some PV antibody was documented also with intracellular domain of both Dsg1 and Dsg3. [195] This finding suggests that anti-desmoglein antibodies can be produced already after the whole desmoglein molecule has been released from the cell membrane of deteriorated keratinocyte into the intercellular space and became available to antigen-presenting cells. In addition, the N-terminal fraction of Dsg3 which is considered to be an immune dominant fraction of the antigen was confirmed in sera of PV patients. [196] Both these findings support the desmoglein sloughing hypothesis.

According to sloughing hypothesis, also other desmosomal cadherins can shed from the cell membrane of deteriorated keratinocytes. Formerly, anti-desmocollin 3 antibody was discovered in PV patients, but in later studies the contrary results were confirmed by ELISA. [197-200] These last findings diminished the role of anti-desmocollin antibody and support the concept that desmocollins are not important autoantigens in pemphigus vulgaris. However, a recent study confirmed the role of desmocollins in desmosome adhesion and showed that the loss of desmocollin 3 in the animal model causes skin blistering. [159] Another recent study confirmed that IgG antibody against desmocollin 3 also induced loss of keratinocyte adhesion *in vitro* in human keratinocyte culture and human epidermis. [201] This finding suggested that an anti-desmocollin 3 antibody contributes to pemphigus vulgaris. This hypothesis was supported by an *in vivo* study on human keratinocytes. The blocking of the desmocollin 3 function was performed by monoclonal antibody against the extracellular domain of desmocollin 3, which led to the formation of intraepidermal blisters and a loss of cell-to-cell adhesion in the keratinocyte culture. [122]

Recent knowledge suggested that the initial trigger in keratinocyte deterioration is sustained by autoantibodies directed at the cell membrane receptors whose binding induces cell shrinkage, the earliest sign of keratinocyte detachment in PV lesions. The most discussed antigens are both acetylcholine receptors, nicotinic and muscarinic, which could be the first target to be assaulted by PV antibodies. [161] The primary involvement hypothesis of autoantibodies against acetylcholin receptors in PV pathogenesis should be confirmed. Another keratinocyte surface antigen pemphaxin, an annexin-like molecule binding acetylcholine, should be simultaneously targeted by autoantibodies and may subsequently induce acantholysis. [162] Additionally, some mitochondrial proteins may also act as antigens. Anti-mitochondrial antibodies seem to be critical. This was provided by studies demonstrating that PV antibodies enter keratinocytes and specially bind to a number of mitochondrial proteins, which is associated with mitochondrial damage, manifested by cytochrome *c* release. Anti-mitochondrial antibodies were pathogenic because their absorption abolished the ability to cause keratinocyte detachment both *in vitro* and *in vivo*, supporting both extrinsic and intrinsic pathways of cell death. [163]

The anti-Dsg1 and anti-Dsg3 antibodies are sensitive markers of pemphigus vulgaris, but their primary role in the pathogenesis of pemphigus vulgaris could be probably overestimated. It is believed that an attack by a constellation of autoantibodies simultaneously targeting several keratinocyte proteins is required to disrupt the integrity of epidermis. The "multiple hit" hypothesis supposes multiple autoantibodies involved in the pathogenesis of pemphigus vulgaris. [202] The first step accounts for anti-acetylcholine receptor antibodies, which trigger acantholysis by weakening the adhesion of neighboring keratinocytes due to inhibition of the control of their polygonal shape, followed by intercellular detachment. This event is followed by a number of immunopathologic and biochemical events leading to acantholysis.

In Vivo and *In Vitro* Models Used in Pemphigus Vulgaris

Classifying a disease as autoimmune requires direct evidence from the transfer of pathogenic antibody or pathogenic T cells and indirect evidence on the reproduction of the autoimmune disease in experimental animals. The first clues on the autoimmune nature of pemphigus vulgaris diseases were provided Beutner, Jordon and co-workers by the demonstration of tissue-bound immunoreactants and serum autoantibodies in 1960s. [203, 204]

Pathomechanisms of blister formation induced by autoantibodies in pemphigus vulgaris have been studied using different *in vitro* and *in vivo* experimental model systems. *In vitro* systems use the keratinocytes culture, human organ culture of the skin, and human skin grafted on mice incubated with autoantibodies, sometimes in the presence of other sera components such as complement or leukocytes. The human organ culture model in pemphigus vulgaris can be used in obtaining information about the mechanism of acantholysis, but is less suitable to reflect biochemical changes concerning molecular pathways, including activation of receptor molecules or phosphorylation state of pathway intermediates. [205] Keratinocyte cultures are the preferred model for biochemical and molecular biological research on acantholysis. Various type of cells are now being used, including normal human epidermal keratinocytes (NHEKs) that are often derived from neonatal foreskin, or from surgical excised skin. Other keratinocyte culture presents HaCaT cells, non-tumorigenic human cell line or squamous cell carcinoma cell line DJM-1. Keratinocyte cultures are mostly used as a monolayer or as reconstituted skin. It was demonstrated that PV antibodies induce acantholysis in cultured human skin after binding to keratinocytes, and they caused destruction of human epidermal cells. [206, 207] Keratinocytes grown in low calcium medium proliferate and in high calcium medium differentiate and form desmosomes and stratify. [208] Keratinocyte culture can be used to research the expression and localization of the PV antigens and other desmosomal adhesion molecules and could help to elucidate acantholysis. [209-212] Human skin grafted on mice is another approach in PV research. There is only limited experience with this model in pemphigus vulgaris. Full-thickness human skin from healthy volunteers was grafted onto

SCID[1] mice and purified IgG fraction from the serum of patients with pemphigus vulgaris and pemphigus foliaceus led to suprabasilar or subcorneal splits in the human grafts, and DIF revealed deposits of IgG in the human grafts. [213] The advantage of the human skin model is that it resembles the real disease in human skin, but cannot fully explain the whole molecular and biochemical activities involved in the pathology of pemphigus.

Animal models have given great insight into the pathology of pemphigus vulgaris. The most respectable *in vivo* model for pemphigus vulgaris exerts mouse models, including different strains of neonatal and adult mice. The experimental data show that after binding to their target antigen, IgG antibodies induce blisters. Anhalt et al. in 1982 provided the first direct evidence that PV antibodies are pathogenic *in vivo*. The authors have used passively transferred IgG fractions from patients with pemphigus vulgaris into neonatal BALB/c mice[2] and demonstrated that PV antibodies induced cutaneous blisters and erosions with the histological, ultrastructural, and immunofluorescence features of pemphigus vulgaris. [170] Subsequently, the pathogenicity of IgG antibodies from patients with sporadic or endemic pemphigus foliaceus was demonstrated using a similar model. [214, 215] An animal model proposing the induction of an autoimmune response in autoimmune blistering diseases was demonstrated by Amagai et al. in 2000. The authors generated an active disease model for pemphigus vulgaris. They used autoantigen-knockout mice lacking Dsg3 (*Dsg3$^{-/-}$*). The *Dsg3$^{-/-}$* mice but not *Dsg3$^{+/-}$*, produced the anti-Dsg3 antibody that bound to native Dsg3, when immunized with recombinant mouse Dsg3. Splenocytes from the immunized Dsg3$^{-/-}$ mice were then transferred into *Rag 2$^{-/-}$* immunodeficient mice that expressed Dsg3. The anti-Dsg3 antibody was produced in the recipient mice and bound to Dsg3 *in vivo,* resulting in deterioration of cell-cell adhesion of keratinocytes. These mice developed the phenotype of pemphigus vulgaris, including oral erosions and suprabasilar acantholysis. [216] The animal model confirmed precisely the pathogenic role of anti-Dsg3 antibody in pemphigus vulgaris Figure 1.6.

Other authors used the same active disease model for pemphigus vulgaris and elucidated the mechanisms of blister formation in pemphigus vulgaris using electron microscopy. The ultrastructural analysis revealed suprabasilar acantholysis, rows of tombstone basilar keratinocytes and half-desmosomes. [217] These findings demonstrated that anti-Dsg3 antibody interfere with the cell-cell adhesion of keratinocytes in the animal PV model. Mahoney et al. in 1999 presented their theories on steric hindrance and desmoglein compensation on normal and DSG3^{null} neonatal mice using passive transfer of PV antibodies. The authors documented that in the areas of epidermis and mucosa that co-express Dsg3 and Dsg1, antibodies against either desmoglein alone do not cause spontaneous blisters, but antibodies against both do. Thus, the anti-Dsg antibody profiles in pemphigus sera and the normal tissue distributions of Dsg1 and Dsg3 determine the sites of blister formation. [146] Step by step the pathogenesis of pemphigus vulgaris was documented using the animal model and concurrently the *in vitro* model as mentioned in the chapter of the molecular mechanism of keratinocytes detachment in pemphigus vulgaris. Takahashi et al. in 2008 demonstrated *in vivo* pathogenicity of Dsg3-reactive T cells at a clonal level in a mouse model for pemphigus vulgaris. Dsg3-reactive T cell lines generated *in vitro* were transferred into Rag-2(-/-) mice

---

[1] SCID mouse (Severe Combined Immune Deficiency) possesses a severe combined immunodeficiency; the humoral and cellular immune systems fail to mature and activate some components of the complement system, and cannot efficiently fight infections, nor reject tumors and transplants.

[2] BALB/c mouse is an albino, laboratory-bred strain of house mouse used in research of immunology and cancer.

with primed B cells derived from Dgs3-imunized Dsg3 (-/-) mice. Some of the cell-line induced anti-Dsg3 antibody and served acantholytic blisters and typical disease phenotype. [218] Tsunoda et al. documented that loss of tolerance against Dsg3 in both B cells and T cells is important for the development of pemphigus vulgaris. They modified an active disease model for pemphigus vulgaris. They used purified T cells and B cells from Dsg3 (-/-), Dsg3 (+/-) or Dsg3 (+/+) mice in various combinations and transferred to Rag-2(-/-) mice. The pathogenic anti-Dsg3 antibody production was observed only with a combination of Dsg3 (-/-) T cells and Dsg3 (-/-) B cells, but not with the other combinations. [219]

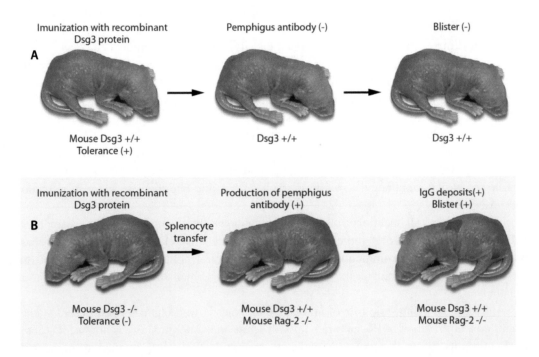

Figure 1.6. Active disease model for autoimmunity in pemphigus vulgaris (According to Amagai et al.).
A- *Dsg3*[+/+] mouse cannot produce pathogenic IgG antibody after immunization with recombinant mouse Dsg3, because it tolerates Dsg3 antigen.
B- *Dsg3*[-/-] mouse after immunization with recombinant mouse Dsg3 induces reactive T cells and B cells to produce antibody against Dsg3. Transferred splenocytes from the immunized *Dsg3*[-/-] mice to *Rag-2*[-/-] produce pathogenic anti-Dgs3 antibody and developed phenotype of pemphigus vulgaris.

There are multiple studies on the animal model that demonstrated the role of PV antibodies. One study demonstrated a time -course of clinical, immunological, ultrastructural, and cytochemical changes in neonatal BALB/c mice after receiving single parenteral injections of PV antibodies. Early epidermal cell detachment was documented using electron microscopy after one hour as a widening of the epidermal intercellular spaces (ICS) and by 6 h the ICS between desmosomes had detached completely. Desmosomes were the last to separate, occurring at 12-18 h. [220] In addition, PV patients' sera, from which the anti-Dsg3 antibody was depleted by immunoabsorption with recombinant protein, no longer induced blister formation in neonatal BALB/c mice. [221]

Also recombinant Dsg3 and Dsg3 various domains were investigated in neonatal mice. This model demonstrates that only EC1 and EC2 extracellular domains of Dsg3 are capable of inducing suprabasilar acantholysis, but when only extracellular domains EC3, EC4 and EC5 were used, acantholysis was not induced. [222] This model indicated that at least one pathogenic epitope, which is sufficient to cause suprabasilar acantholysis in neonatal mice is located on domains EC1 and EC2. A recent study detected that PV antibodies targeted the EC1 and EC2 domains of Dsg3 in regions that are involved in *cis*-adhesive interactions. [223] The study was performed in a passive transfer model in neonatal mice and also on keratinocytes monolayers *in vitro*. These findings identified the *cis*-adhesive interface of Dsg3 as the immunodominant region targeted by pathogenic antibodies.

Shimizu et al. analyzed the ultrastructural localization of *in vivo*-bound antibody to Dsg3 during the acantholysis process using post-embedding immunoelectron microscopy. [224] The study revealed that within the acantholytic areas, there were abundant split-desmosomes with intermediate filaments inserted into the desmosomal attachment plaques. These desmosome extracellular regions were covered with anti-Dsg3 antibody and were associated with desmoplakin in their cytoplasmic attachment plaques. No apparent split-desmosomes free of IgG antibody were observed, suggesting that Dsg3 was not depleted from the desmosome before the start of acantholysis *in vivo*. [224] These findings indicate that anti-Dsg3 antibody can directly invade Dsg3 in desmosomes *in vivo* and cause the subsequent desmosome separation leading to blister formation in pemphigus vulgaris. Anti-Dsg3 antibody caused desmosomal splitting without intermediate filament retraction at the apical surfaces of basilar keratinocytes, while on their lateral side intermediate filament retraction was observed. [224]

The results of all mentioned *in vivo* investigations above suggest that the pemphigus vulgaris mice model is a representative experimental model representing the disease phenotype from both an immunological and ultrastructural point of view. In addition, this model can help to elucidate the immunomolecular mechanism of blister formation in acantholysis.

Although the pathogenic role of anti-Dsg antibodies is well characterized, recent studies identified a novel target of PV autoimmunity. It seems that autoimmunity is not just restricted to desmogleins. From this point of view, the scenario of blister formation in pemphigus vulgaris after the binding of autoantibodies to keratinocytes remained largely unclear. All the mentioned studies were focused on "primary" autoantigens desmogleins, predominantly Dsg3. Other desmosome antigens including plakoglobin, desmoplakin and desmocollins are the targets for specific autoantibodies as mentioned in the chapter on autoantigens and autoantibodies. Various anti-keratinocyte antibodies may concur to cause blistering by acting synergistically with anti-Dsg antibodies, as has been described through the "multiple hit" hypothesis. [202] The mice model was used to demonstrate that additionally to Dsg1 and Dsg3, other keratinocyte antigens can be targeted by PV antibodies causing clinical phenotype of pemphigus vulgaris. The authors used PV antibodies after absorption of anti-Dsg1 and anti-Dsg3 antibody using rDsg1 and rDsg3. These "clean" PV antibodies caused skin blisters in $Dsg3^{null}$ mice and "balding" $Dsg3^{bal}/Dsg3^{bal}$ mice[3]. Pemphigus vulgaris-like suprabasilar acantholysis indicated that pemphigus vulgaris phenotype can be induced without anti-Dsg3 and anti-Dsg1 antibodies and may induce skin blistering formation. [225] This experiment supported the hypothesis that additionally other target antigen than desmogleins are responsible for binding PV antibodies and may cause acantholysis.

---

[3] $Dsg3^{bal}/Dsg3^{bal}$ mice carries a spontaneous null mutation in Dsg3.

In addition, the active disease mouse model for pemphigus vulgaris can be used as a tool to evaluate various immunosuppressive therapeutic strategies. The efficacy of an evaluated drug can be measured by the level of production of anti-Dsg3 antibody, body weight loss that reflects the severity of oral erosions, and PV score that reflects the extent of skin lesions. [226] Another model, neonatal BALB/c mice, was used to demonstrate mitochondria-mediated intrinsic apoptosis by sera from patients with pemphigus vulgaris. The mitochondrial protecting drugs nicotinamide, minocycline, and cyclosporine A exhibited uniform protective effects. [227]

In conclusion, experimental data have been mostly obtained by using PV antibody purified from patient sera, which contain not only antibodies against a variety of different epitopes of Dsg3 and Dsg1, but also other antibodies against other antigens of desmosomal plaque or non-desmosomal antigens of other origin, especially from the keratinocyte surface. However, anti-Dsg antibodies are considered to be a diagnostic hallmark for pemphigus vulgaris despite not always reflecting the disease activity and maybe not always being pathogenic. According to new knowledge, they probably play the role of witness in the pathogenesis of pemphigus vulgaris rather than the role of causative inducer of acantholysis.

REGULATION OF PEMPHIGUS VULGARIS AUTOIMMUNITY

Autoimmunity is a normal event. Any individual develops immune reactions against numerous self antigens, but this condition only rarely leads to autoimmune disease. Autoimmune disease results from an aberration of this normal phenomenon. [228] The etiology of this switch is deemed multifactorial with the final common pathway being the loss of normal self-tolerance in a particular organ, or group of organs. In pemphigus vulgaris, the target organ of autoimmunity is the stratified squamous epithelium. Genetic, environmental, hormonal and immunological factors are considered important in the development of autoimmune disease. Among them, HLA genes are believed to be the most important predisposition factors in the pathogenesis of pemphigus vulgaris, because they serve the autoantigen to immune competent cells. Thus, antigen presentation induces the autoimmunity event. The other loci probably participate in an additive or epistatic manner.

The basis of autoimmunity in pemphigus vulgaris has been studied on the assumption that Dsg1 and Dsg3 antibodies solely induce autoimmunity. Recent studies discovered various antigens that significantly might participate in the pathogenesis of pemphigus vulgaris. From this point of view, the autoimmunity event remains unrecognized. Autoreactive T cells are thought to play a central role in the pathogenesis of pemphigus vulgaris. Recently, in the spotlight is a new subset of Th17 cells producing interleukin -17 (IL-17). Emerging data refer that Th17 cells play an important role in host defense and are highly pro-inflammatory. In addition, Th17 cells with specificity for self-antigens lead to severe autoimmunity in various animal models. [229] A high IL-17 expression has also been detected in the target tissue during the progression of various organ-specific autoimmune diseases, such as multiple sclerosis, rheumatoid arthritis, systemic lupus erythematosus and psoriasis. [230-233] It was referred that the development and maintenance of Th17 cells have been linked to IL-23, a key initiating cytokine in the development of autoimmunity. [234] A crucial role was proposed for the IL-23/IL-17 axis in mediating tissue inflammation and autoimmunity in various organ-specific autoimmune diseases, as well as in pemphigus vulgaris. [235-238]

The next new field in investigation of pemphigus vulgaris pathogenesis is B cells. Recently, it has been described that B cells are able to negatively regulate cellular immune responses and inflammation. Previously, B cells had been regarded for their capacity to produce antibody. However, recent advances demonstrated that B cells also release a broad variety of cytokines. They are classified into subsets according to their cytokine production. One functional subset, regulatory B cells (Breg), has been functionally defined to contribute to the maintenance of peripheral tolerance and homeostasis. [239] Breg cells inhibit the excessive inflammatory responses in autoimmune disease by their ability to produce IL-10, which inhibits proinflammatory cytokines and promotes regulatory T cell differentiation. Breg cells with the capacity to produce IL-10 have been named B10 cells. B10 cells exclusively produce IL-10 and are the predominant B cell source of IL-10. [240] The function of Breg cells was documented in various organ-specific autoimmune diseases, including systemic lupus erythematosus, rheumatoid arthritis, multiple sclerosis and Graves´ disease, while with pemphigus vulgaris it was only in two studies. [241-247]

The relevance of anti-Dgs3 antibody in pemphigus vulgaris is well defined. Since the autoimmunity in pemphigus vulgaris is mediated by autoantibodies, it is postulated that T cells participate in the pathogenesis of the disease in the stages leading to production of pathogenic autoantibodies.

Antibody production by B cells requires the participation of T helper-(Th) cells in T cell-dependent antibody responses. After antigen-driven activation of T cells, they induce to secrete cytokines that are crucial in switching of B cell antibody production.

According to sole Dsg autoimmunity, the most important event is the Th1 and Th2 recognition of Dsg3 peptides restricted by HLA DRB1*04:02 and or HLA DQB1*05:03. [248, 249] The Dsg3-specific T cells expressed a memory T cell phenotype and Th2 cytokine profile that modulate the pathogenic autoantibody response in pemphigus vulgaris. [250, 251] HLA allele restriction was additionally documented in transgenic PV model mice of hyplotype HLA class II. In the study, a class II tetramer -based detection system uses HLA DRB1* 04:02 tetramers loaded with previously identified T cell epitopes of Dsg3. The authors documented human Dsg-reactive T cells in patients with pemphigus vulgaris. [252]

The role of various HLA alleles for increasing susceptibility to pemphigus vulgaris is mainly attributed to the electric charge of Dsg3-derived epitopes and their ability to bind to distinct HLA alleles upon recognition by autoreactive T cells. [253] Figure 1.7.

Molecules that code HLA DR1*04:02 differ from other HLA-DR4 molecules by the presence of a negative charge at amino acid residue 71 and 70 in the β chain, which is a critical binding motif for T cell peptides. Several T cell reactive to epitopes of Dsg3 have been identified that carry a positively charged amino acid (mostly lysine or arginine) at relative position 4 (p4), which serves as an anchor motif to the negatively charged p4 pocket formed by residues at position 70 and 71 of DRB1*04:02. Thus, DRB1*04:02 shapes the fine specificity of the T cell against a limited set of Dsg3 epitopes that fulfill the binding criteria of this specific HLA class II molecule. Modified from ref. [254]

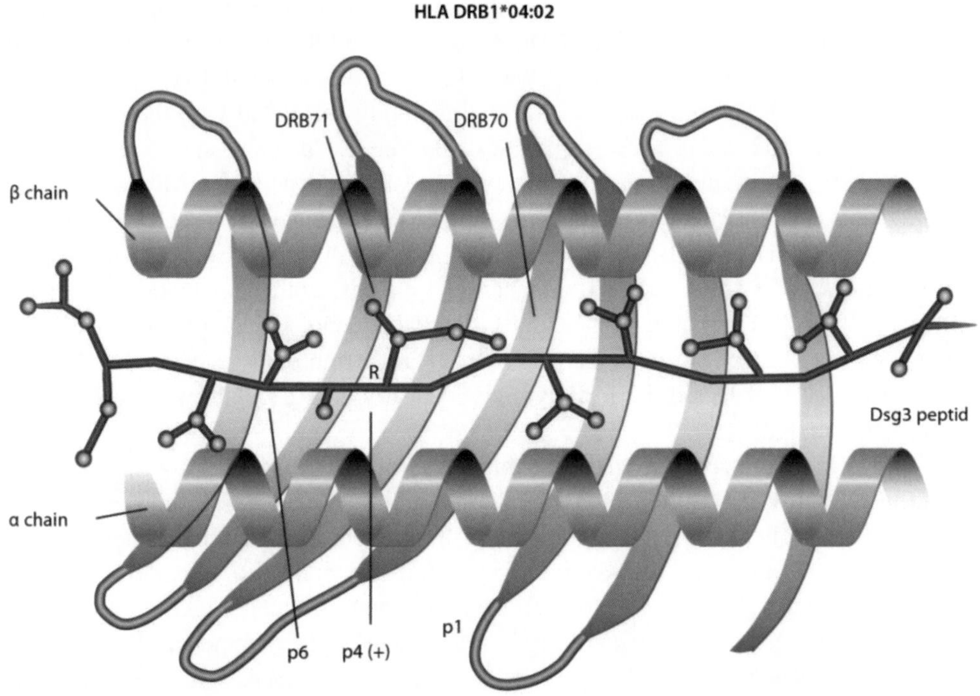

HLA DRB1*04:02

Figure 1.7. Algorithm for HLA class II-Desmoglein 3 interaction in pemphigus vulgaris.

HLA DRB1*04:02 and DQB1*05:03 were found to have a similar avidity for the binding of Dsg3, but at different locations with HLA DRB1*04:02 binding to peptides derived from the extracellular Dsg domain and DQB1*05:03 binding to COOH-terminal Dsg3 subdomains, suggesting multiple interactions of Dsg3 peptides with the restricting HLA class II alleles. [255] The study model data strongly indicates that multiple initial epitopes may be responsible for both disease initiation and progression. It remains to be determined which proportion of predicted DRB1*04:02 and DQB1*05:03 binders are competent to stimulate pemphigus vulgaris associated alleles and autoreactive T cells. [255]

The loss of self-tolerance against Dsg3 in both T cells and B cells is required for efficient production of anti-Dsg3 antibody. Dsg3-specific B cells and memory B cells were detected in peripheral blood from patients with pemphigus vulgaris and suggested that HLA class II restriction collaboration between Dsg3-reactive T cells and Dsg3-reactive B cells is important for anti-Dsg3antibody production. [256] The PV model mice were used to confirm Dsg3-reactive T cells and Dsg3-reactive B cells. Pathogenic anti-Dsg3 antibody production was observed only with a combination of Dsg3$^{-/-}$ T cells and Dsg3$^{-/-}$ B cells. [219] Furthermore, PV model mice and subsequent *in vitro* analysis were used to identify cytokine production by Dsg3-reactive T cells. IL-4 promoted anti-Dsg3 antibody production by Dsg3-reactive B cells. Additionally, the block with IL-4R in vivo suppressed anti-Dsg3 antibody production. [218] Results of previous studies suggest that loss of tolerance against Dsg3 in both B cells and T cells is required for development of the autoimmune condition of pemphigus vulgaris and indicates a pathogenic role of IL-4. An *in vitro* study evaluated the quantity of Dsg3-reactive T cells in patients with acute onset, chronic active and remittent pemphigus vulgaris. Dsg3-reactive Th2 cells were detected at similar frequencies in all type of pemphigus vulgaris, while the number of Dsg3-reactive Th1 cells exceeded those of Th2 cells in chronic active pemphigus vulgaris. In contrast, healthy carriers of pemphigus vulgaris associated HLA class II alleles, DRB1*04:02 and DQB1*05:03, exhibited exclusively Dsg3-reactive Th1 responses, while healthy carriers of other HLA class II alleles did not. [257] Another study observed that the titers of serum anti-Dsg3 antibody correlated with the proportion of Dsg3-reactive Th1/Th2 cells. These results strongly suggest that the appearance of Dsg3-reactive Th2 cells is restricted to patients with active pemphigus vulgaris. Moreover, specific HLA class II alleles prevalent in pemphigus vulgaris are critical for T cell recognition of Dsg3 in PV patients and Dsg3-responsive healthy individuals. Likewise, Dsg1-reactive Th1 and Th2 cells were found in similar frequencies in patients with pemphigus foliaceus and healthy controls. [258] Hertl et al. demonstrated that PV patients with active disease exhibited *in vitro* CD4$^+$ T cell responses to the EC1-5 of Dsg3. Furthermore, Dsg3-reactive CD4$^+$ T cell responses were also detected in healthy individuals with HLA alleles associated with pemphigus vulgaris. [259]

Another study demonstrated that the blockade of the CD40/CD154 interaction by treatment with anti-CD154 monoclonal antibody inhibited the production of anti-Dsg3 antibody and subsequently the development of the pemphigus vulgaris phenotype in PV model mice. [260] Interaction between antigen-specific T cells and B cells via their co-stimulatory molecules is required for efficient antibody production. One of these co-stimulatory molecules, CD154 (CD40 ligand; a B cell surface molecule), is expressed transiently on activated T cells. Interaction of these molecules leads to proliferation and differentiation of B cells. [261] The findings of the last study therefore indicate that the CD40/CD154 interaction is essential to induce the production of pathogenic PV antibodies and that the blockade with anti-CD154 monoclonal antibody may restore tolerance against Dsg3 and prevent the development of pemphigus vulgaris.

Recently, the role of Th17 cells is considered to be a spotlight in the investigation of PV autoimmunity. The IL-23/IL-17 axis has been identified as a major factor involved in the pathogenesis of several organ-specific autoimmune disease, including pemphigus vulgaris. Xue et al. documented that the PV lesions overexpressed both IL-23 and IL-17 in correlation with Th17 cells and CD163 cells. [238] The last molecule is considered a surface marker of macrophages. In accordance with previous results, the higher expression of Th17 cells in PV lesions compared to control was detected also in another study. [262] Taken together, Th17 cells and the IL-23/IL-17 axis are suggested as playing an important role in the pathogenesis of pemphigus vulgaris. Interestingly, macrophages (CD163+ cells), which are suggested to play an important role in pathogenesis of psoriasis may also be involved in the pathogenesis of pemphigus vulgaris. In contrast, it was referred that the IL-17 presence in PV lesions correlated neither with anti-Dsg3 antibody serum levels nor with the clinical severity of pemphigus vulgaris. [262, 263] On the other hand, *in vitro* studies on epidermal keratinocytes observed autoreactive cytotoxic T cells that are sensitized to putative keratinocyte antigens in PV patients. [264]The result of this study was in accordance with the results of CD8 deficient PV model mice in pemphigus vulgaris. [265] Taken together, these results suggest that cytotoxic T cells may play a role in the pathogenesis of pemphigus vulgaris.

The Role of Regulatory T and B Cells in Pemphigus Vulgaris

Regulatory T cells (Tregs) play an imperative key role in the maintenance of immunologic self-tolerance and homeostasis. However, they negatively control a variety of physiological and pathological immune responses. Tregs exert a dominant effect in autoimmunity controlling. Treg are the naturally occurring CD4+CD25+ cells, which express the transcription factor Foxp3 (forkhead box P3). [266] Several reports confirmed a few presences of Tregs in healthy skin and a little higher in PV lesional skin, although the difference was not significant. [267] The frequency of Treg in the peripheral blood of PV patients, however, was significantly decreased in the number of Tregs compared with healthy control. [268] Consistent with these results, an increased number of Tr1 cells specific for Dsg3 were found in healthy carriers of HLA class II alleles associated with pemphigus vulgaris. [269] Functionally mature Tregs are specialized for the suppressive function that inhibits the activation of Th cells. While the induction of Treg suppressive activity is specific and requires antigenic stimulation through a T cell receptor, the suppression exerted by Tregs is antigenic nonspecific. [270] Tregs are produced in the thymus and can also be induced from naive T cells in the periphery. Tregs represents up to 10% of peripheral CD4+ T cells and operate in a cell contact-dependent and non-antigen -specific manner as they are presumably activated *in vitro*. [272] Various Tregs can participate in distinct mechanisms to collaboratively regulate the duration and intensity of immune responses. [272] Among those, the most prominent is type 1 Treg (Tr1), which has been employed to be induced upon antigen exposure under certain tolerogenic conditions. Tr1 cells produce cytokines IL-10 and TGF-β. [273] Defects in Tregs activity have been referred in various human organ-specific autoimmune diseases including pemphigus vulgaris. Recently, it was referred that Dsg3-reactive Tr1 is predominant in healthy individuals with PV-associated HLA class II alleles, HLA DRB1*04:02 and DQB1*05:03, and only in less than 20% of PV patients. However, Dsg3-reactive T cells were recently found in both PV patients and healthy individuals with PV -associated HLA class II alleles. [269] These findings suggest that Dsg3-reactive Tr1 may be critically involved in the maintenance and restoration of peripheral tolerance against Dsg3 in healthy individuals, as well as in PV patients. [269] In concordance with the former findings, the portion of Treg cell population was severely reduced, approximately ten times less in PV patients than in controls. [274] These results demonstrate that a deficiency of Tregs in PV patient´s peripheral blood is not accompanied by a decrease in Tregs in PV lesions. Thus, the decrease in peripheral blood may result from the accumulation of Tregs in skin lesions and draining lymph nodes. [275] Another explanation may be the fact that the deficiency in Trg1 cells is directly related to the loss of tolerance against Dsg3 and consistent with the detection of low peripheral Treg cells in patients with active pemphigus vulgaris, and that they both regulatory T cells cooperate in loss of the tolerance in pathogenesis of pemphigus vulgaris. PV model mice demonstrated that Treg controlled the anti-Dsg3 antibody production as follows: adoptively transferred Tregs suppressed the antibody production in a dose-dependent manner and the depletion of endogenous Tregs augmented the antibody production. [276] These findings are in accordance with previous studies that showed that Tregs have a suppressive role in antigen-specific antibody production and their down-regulation leads to increased antibody production. In addition, the loss of tolerance against Dsg3 in pemphigus vulgaris is presumably dependent on a deficiency of both Treg and Tr1cells, accompanied by other cells involved in immune processes. Arakawa et al.

referred that pemphigus vulgaris lesions contained both Treg expressing Foxp3 factor and IL-17 produced by Th17 cells. [275] However, it was referred that local findings were not found in concordance with the serum level of IL-17. [262] Figure 1.8 shows the hypothetical scheme of immune dysregulation in pemphigus vulgaris. Modified from ref. [254]

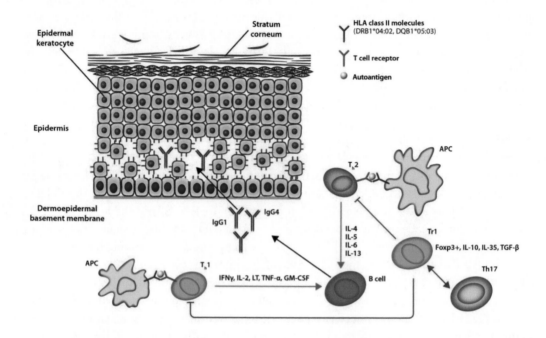

Figure 1.8. Hypothetical scheme of immune dysregulation in pemphigus vulgaris.

Pemphigus vulgaris is the prototype of an autoantibody-mediated autoimmune disorder. IgG production by autoreactive B cells is regulated by Dsg3- and Dsg1-reactive Th1 and Th2 cells. The Dsg3-reactive Th cells recognize epitopes of Dsg3 ectodomain in association with the HLA class II alleles HLA DRB1*04:02 and DQB1*05:03 presented by APCs. Tregs may be critical in maintaining peripheral B cell tolerance to Dsg3. Proinflammatory Th17 cells influence the pathogenesis of pemphigus vulgaris. Abbreviations: APC, antigen presenting cells; IL, interleukin. Modified from Ref. [254]

Recently, regulatory B cells (Bregs) have been functionally defined to contribute to the maintenance of peripheral tolerance and homeostasis. [239] After stimulation, Bregs produce IL-10 (B10 cells), which inhibits pro-inflammatory cytokines and promotes Treg differentiation. [240] The first study about B cell response in patients with pemphigus vulgaris after rituximab therapy observed differences in the Breg cell population. PV patients in complete remission revealed a fourfold higher number of B10 cells than those in incomplete remission. [246] Another study referred elevated Breg cells in periphery circulation in patients with pemphigus vulgaris, but the B10 cell possessed a defective regulatory function on Th1 cells. [247] The role of the Breg cell and correlation between T cells and B cells in the maintenance of peripheral tolerance and homeostasis remains to be determined.

In conclusion, autoimmunity in pemphigus vulgaris is developing according to the rules of antibody mediated autoimmune diseases. Dsg-1 and Dsg3-reactive T cells are considered to be exclusively leading cells in cooperation with B cells that line the anti-Dsg1 and anti-Dsg3 antibodies production. Treg cells, which are required for maintenance of peripheral tolerance and homeostasis, are higher in healthy individuals with HLA class II alleles associated with pemphigus vulgaris than in PV patients with active disease. A decrease in Treg cells in peripheral blood of PV patients does not validate the postulated deficiency of the immunosuppressive activity, because Treg cells are present in PV lesions. The role of other regulatory cells such as Breg cells in the autoimmunity of pemphigus vulgaris remains to be determined, as well as the putative interplay between Treg cells and Th17 cells. In addition the role of autoreactive T cells and B cells against autoantigens involved in the "multiple -hit "hypothesis should be investigated.

MOLECULAR MECHANISMS OF KERATINOCYTE DETACHMENT IN PEMPHIGUS VULGARIS

Acantholysis is due to alteration of the adhesive property of desmogleins with consequent loss of desmosomal function. Several hypotheses have been tried to explain the mechanism of pemphigus vulgaris acantholysis. The classical explanation for suprabasal acantholysis in pemphigus vulgaris is that antibodies to Dsg3 and Dsg1 block the function of these two adhesion molecules by steric hindrance or by altering their structure, leading directly to desmosomal dissociation. [277-280] The restriction of acantholysis to the basal layer is explained by Dsg3 being expressed predominantly in the deeper epidermal layers and Dsg1 in the more superficial layers. According to the compensation theory, blisters occur only in deep epidermal layers in pemphigus vulgaris and only in superficial layers in pemphigus foliaceus. However, the steric hindrance hypothesis cannot be a fully satisfactory explanation, as acantholysis does not appear to be triggered by loss of adhesion between desmosomes and its restriction to the basal layer in pemphigus vulgaris appears to involve other factors than Dsg compensation. In addition, the explanation has been challenged by numerous reports showing activation of specific signalling pathways in keratinocytes exposed to anti-Dsg antibody. The steric hindrance hypothesis is based on numerous assumptions that the binding of anti-Dsg antibody in the epidermis is limited to desmosomes, as it was confirmed by passive transfer of PV antibody recognizing uniquely Dsg3 and Dsg1 in pemphigus vulgaris model mice. [221, 281] Generally, desmoglein molecules are predominantly localized to desmosomes, but the binding of PV antibody extends well beyond the desmosomes decorating the entire surface of keratinocytes. [282] Furthermore, pemphigus foliaceus (PF) antibody has been shown to cause the dissociation of keratinocytes by involving of autoantibody-triggered cellular signalling pathways, without blocking Dsg1 homophilic transinteraction resulting in the destabilization of Dsg1-based adhesive sites and desmosomes. [283] It was demonstrated that anti-Dsg3 antibody in pemphigus vulgaris directly inhibit Dsg3 transinteraction, whereas in contrast, anti-Dsg1antibody in pemphigus vulgaris and pemphigus foliaceus reduce Dsg1 transinteraction not directly, but rather indirectly via cellular mechanisms. [284] It is suggested that the direct inhibition of Dsg3 transinteraction or activation of cell-signalling mechanisms may not be mutually exclusive, but rather act in concern in pemphigus pathogenesis. Moreover, it is unlikely that the direct inhibition of Dsg3 transinteraction alone is responsible for desmosomal splitting and acantholysis in pemphigus vulgaris.

A recent study proposed the adhesion receptor signaling through integrins, but also cadherines, to transmit extracellular stimuli in an outside-in mode to inversely modulate EGFR signalling and to ensure cell survival. Thus, in pemphigus vulgaris non-Dsg molecules are targeted by pathogenic PV antibody in the interdesmosomal areas, which is interpreted as targeting of Dsg3 located outside of the desmosomes. [285] The alternative Dsg3 alteration hypotheses possess a broad spectrum of outside-in signals elicited due to the binding of PV antibody to keratinocytes emanating exclusively from Dsg3. Therefore, Dsg3 is considered to act as both adhesion molecule and signal transmitter. [285-287]

According to Grando, the following hypothetical chain of events is speculated as follows: 1/ PV antibody signalling is initiated by ligation of the nonfunctional pool of Dsg3 outside of the desmosome; 2/ when ligated by an autoantibody, these putative nonfunctional Dsg3 molecules, either membrane associated or internalized or both, send signals that impair Dsg3 trafficking into and out of desmosome ; 3/the supposedly impaired Dsg trafficking specifically depletes Dsg3 from desmosome without changes in other functional proteins. [150]

The whole pemphigus vulgaris IgG fraction, rather than anti-Dsg3 antibody purified from patients with active pemphigus vulgaris was used to discover biologic responses in the pathogenesis of pemphigus vulgaris. Recently, a biologic effect was referred of PV antibody on keratinocytes expressing the Ds3 molecules, whose epitopes are responsible for pathogenic binding were hidden due to cell pre-incubation with the anti-Dsg3 monoclonal antibody AK23[4] that decreased the amount of Dsg3 in cultured keratinocytes. The keratinocytes demonstrated binding PV antibody-like signalling. [288] Therefore, the depletion of Dsg3 is suggested to be a secondary event resulting from inside-out signalling caused by a keratinocyte response to the pathogenic PV antibodies that deliver an initial insult. With the in vitro model, the anti-Dsg3 monoclonal antibody AK23 to a single extracellular domain of Dsg3 can deplete desmosomes of Dsg3, leaving Dsg2 and desmoplakins and cell-cell adhesion. [289] These results suggest that the anti-Dsg3 antibody itself cannot completely eliminate the desmosomal adhesive function. However, loss of Dsg3 from desmosome does weaken the adhesive strength of this structure. In this event, the primary role should be played by the anti-PERP[5] antibody in the depletion of Dsg3. An observation suggested that the binding of PV antibody triggers the internalization of PERP, which enhances the depletion of desmosomal Dgs3 and intercellular adhesion defects. [290] Other studies of pemphigus vulgaris referred that PV antibodies act via plakoglobin to abolish the c-Myc suppression required for both maintenance of epidermal stem cells in their niche and controlled differentiation along the epidermal lineage. [128, 291] These data identify plakoglobin as a potent modulator of epithelial homeostasis via its role as a key suppressor of c-Myc.

---

[4] AK23 monoclonal antibody recognizes residues 1-161(the amino-terminal portion of the extracellular domain) of Dsg3 and cross-reacts with human (h) Dsg3 in human epidermal keratinocytes or human squamous cell carcinoma cell line (DJM-1).

[5] PERP[2] is a p53-regulated gene, a tetraspan membrane protein that belongs to the tetraspan family. Members of the tetraspan family play central or regulatory roles in a wide variety of physiological processes through their interaction with other membrane proteins. PERP was originally identified as an apoptosis-associated target of the p53 tumor suppressor. In epidermis, PERP plays an important role in epithelial integrity through a function at the desmosome. A PERP deficient mouse exhibits blistering in oral mucosa and skin. [293]

The exclusive role of anti-Dsg1 and Dsg3 antibodies in pemphigus vulgaris pathogenesis, which causes steric hindrance at the adhesion points of keratinocytes, has been largely reevaluated. The pathologic outcome of PV antibody-induced signalling is induction of the apoptotic and/or oncotic pathways, associated with the collapse of the cytoskeleton, because of keratin filament retraction and actin reorganization, cell shrinkage, caused by cell volume decrease, and finally, cell-cell dyshesion (acantholysis).

The outside-in signalling of PV antibody can be evoked through both cholinergic receptors and desmosomal proteins, as well as other yet unknown antigen or receptors ligated on the cell membrane of keratinocyte by an array of PV antibodies other than anti-Dsg IgG produced in each patient, as explicated by the "multiple –hit" hypothesis. [201] It is suggested that cholinergic receptors play an important role in inducing acantholysis. The major downstream signalling event is considered to result from activation of cholinergic receptors expressed in keratinocytes. The principal signalling event is triggered due to antibody interference with the physiological control of keratinocyte growth and differentiation, shape and adhesion and motility. [292]

It is important to elucidate the outside-in signaling pathways mediated by PV antibody and so understand pathogenesis in pemphigus vulgaris. The *in vitro* and *in vivo* studies would like to discover the complexity of PV antibody signalling, and also clearly demonstrate the therapeutic potential of kinase inhibitors and pathway modifiers. PV antibody-dependent acantholysis in experimental animals is improved by inhibitors of phospholipase C, protein kinase C, m TOR, p38MAPK, other tyrosine kinases, calmodulin and cholinergic agonists. [294, 296, 298] The triggering events, however, remain obscure. The outside-in signalling elicited due to the binding of PV antibodies to keratinocytes proceeds via different pathways, consistent with simultaneous ligation of several types of cell surface receptors by distinct antibodies produced by pemphigus patients.

The critical moment in the hierarchy of signaling events leading to acantholysis is the kinase activation. The activation of tyrosine kinases receptor (TKRs) at an early step of PV antibody-induced signalling suggested that such receptors are either novel specific targets in pemphigus vulgaris or just a result of the collateral damage produced by PV antibody binding to the keratinocyte cell membrane, or both. Frusic-Zlotkin et al. documented that activation of cell surface receptor EGFR by PV antibody was followed by its internalization on keratinocyte culture *in vitro*. [297] EGFR activation is considered to be a pivotal for intracellular apoptotic signal transduction via ERK/c-Jun pathways, leading to apoptosis induction (FasR pathway), which later led to major cell-cell separation (acantholysis) and cell death. [298] The activation of p38 MAPK is a late signalling step associated with collapse of the cytoskeleton and disassembly of desmosomes cased by upstream events involving c-Src kinase[6] and EGFR kinase. The early signalling events were triggered predominantly by non-Dsg PV antibodies, and involved activation of Src and EGFR kinase associated with the collapse of the cytoskeleton. Anti-Dsg1 and -Dsg3 antibodies contributed predominantly to the pathologic event associated with p38 MAPK activation, a late signalling step, linked to keratinocyte apoptosis. [299] To dissect out the signalling pathways originating from Dsg1/ Dsg3 and from those elicited due to ligation of non-Dsg antigens, authors used keratinocyte culture with the knocked-down expression of the *DSG1* and/or *DSG3* genes by small

---

[6] c-Src kinase is a protein encoded by the cellular counterpart of the translation product of the *src* gene of Rous sarcoma virus.

interfering RNA (siRNA). The earliest acantholytic events appeared to be triggered by non-Dsg antibodies. [299] Activation of EGFR was followed by phosphorylation of its downstream substrates, MAP kinase and transcription factor c-Jun, and internalization of EGFR. These observations were confirmed by pharmacological inactivation of the EGRF and MAP kinase activities, by use of their specific inhibitors that blocked PV antibody -induced phosphorylation of EGFR, MAP and c-Jun and cellular apoptosis, measured by flow cytometry and caspase 3 activity. [297] Activation of PKC through the phosphatidylcholine-specific phospholipase C pathway is also one of the earliest actions in PV antibody-induced acantholysis. [300] These observations revealed an evident array of interconnected signalling cascades emanating from different cell surface antigens simultaneously targeted by a constellation of patients´ anti-keratinocyte antibodies that trigger acantholysis and keratinocyte death in pemphigus vulgaris.

Alterations in desmosome assembly and disassembly are thought to compromise desmosome function in pemphigus vulgaris. PV antibodies target the extracellular domain of Dsg3 or both Dsg3 and Dsg1. Recently, several studies demonstrated that PV antibody aberrantly induce clustering of desmoglein autoantigens. [301, 302]. This event leads to degradation and loss of Dsg3 steady state levels at the plasma membrane, resulting in desmosome disassembly, keratin filament retraction, and a significantly compromised ability of keratinocyte sheets to resist mechanical stress. [303, 289] Polyclonal PV antibodies are responsible for aberrant cell surface clustering and endocytosis of Dsg3, through a clathrin- and dynamin[7]-independent endocytic pathway. [304] Furthermore, PV antibody-induced internalization occurs via a membrane raft[8]-mediated pathway, indicating that Dsg3 raft association provides a means for desmosome regulation. They are also known as lipid rafts or detergent resistant membranes. The membrane rafts are highly ordered microdomains within the plasma membrane. Individual raft domains can cluster to form larger, ordered domains that function as a platform for a variety of cellular processes such as signalling, endocytosis and membrane organization. [305] It was documented that membrane rafts also regulate the dynamics of desmosome assembly and disassembly and thereby modulate normal keratinocyte adhesion, as well as keratinocyte responses to PV antibodies. [306]

Saito et al. demonstrated that the endocytosis of Dsg3 occurred in a p38 MAPK-dependent manner. [301] In contrast, pathogenic monoclonal anti-Dsg3 antibody causes loss of adhesion in a p38 MAPK-independent fashion that is most likely dependent on the ability of this antibody to sterically hinder Dsg3 adhesive interaction. [301] The IgG-induced clustering of the desmoglein autoantigens underlies the granular IgG deposition in patient skin. In pemphigus foliaceus and in mucocutaneous pemphigus vulgaris, Dsg1 clustering but not Dsg3 clustering, correlates with nonacantholytic intercellular widening between desmosomes. [302] In pemphigus vulgaris, the desmogleins become sequestered from desmosomal components which fit in with the desmoglein nonassembly depletion hypothesis, indicating that targeted conjunctional desmogleins are no longer available to be incorporated

---

[7] Clathrin-dynamin mediated endocytosis is the endocytic portal into cells the cargo of which is packaged into vesicles with the aid of a clathrin coat and the latter with dynamin-mediated scission. It is fundamental to signal transduction, neurotransmission and the regulation of many plasma membrane activities and so is essential to higher eukaryotic life. Some modules can be used in other pathways according to cell specificity and adaptability.

[8] Membrane raft are small (10-200 nm) heterogenous, highly dynamic, sterol- and sphingolipid-enriched domains that compartmentalize the cellular process. Small raft can sometimes be stabilized to form a larger platform through protein-protein and protein-lipid interaction. [306]

into desmosomes and this leads to disturbed assembly, and Dsg-depleted desmosomes. [302] PV antibody triggers two major events after ligation to Dsg3 at the cell surface. At first, PV antibodies cause the disassembly of desmosomes at or near the cell surface, and also cause the retraction of keratin intermediate filaments from lateral cell-cell borders. Secondly, PV antibodies trigger the co-endocytosis of Dsg3 and plakoglobin, leading to the delivery of Dsg3 to the lysosomal compartment and a dramatic decrease in Dsg3 protein levels. [307] Taken together, PV antibodies may not only disrupt desmosomal mediated adhesion, but may also trigger the disruption of protein complex within the desmosomal plaque. Thus, PV antibody binding to Dsg3 triggers a cascade of events leading to the disruption of desmosomes and the loss of adhesion molecules on the cell surface. [303, 308]

Independent of localization in desmosomes, desmosomal cadherins also appear "extradesmosomal" in the membrane connected to actin filaments. Extradesmosomal cadherins interact with signaling molecules and so are involved in adhesion-dependent and adhesion-independent outside-in signaling rather than being crucial for intercellular cohesion only. [285, 286] Several studies indicated that the pool of anti-keratinocyte antibodies produced by pemphigus vulgaris patients contains anti-Dsg1 and anti-Dsg3 antibodies, and non-Dsg antibodies. The non-Dsg antibodies are the major contributors to early signalling events. Early activation of the Src/EGFR kinase and protein kinase C -dependent pathway is evidently pathogenic because it leads to acantholysis, and a late activation of p38MAPK is secondary to cell detachment. [297, 309] The Src-dependent cascade is another member also responsible for keratinocyte shrinkage (cell volume reduction). A time course experiment demonstrated that the activities of Src and EGFR kinase peak at 30-60 min after exposure of PV antibodies, suggesting that engagement of Src/ EGFR kinase is a critical step that generates signals from ligated antigens to the intracellular effectors. The keratinocyte shrinkage became significant at 120 min and keratin aggregation at 240 min, with an increase of TUNEL positivity at 360 min. [299] The cytoskeletal collapse has been reported as an early event that precedes visible separation. [310, 311] The timing of acantholysis appears that of pemphigus vulgaris IgG antibody-induced phosphorylation of adhesive molecules and structural proteins leads to weakening of intercellular junctions and collapse of the cytoskeleton. [150]

Several studies referred the binding of PV antibody to the surface of epidermal cells in early and established lesions. Desmosomes do not split, but they separate when the intercellular spaces are already widened followed by the separation of desmosomal junctions as the last event. [312, 313] The binding of PV antibody triggers signalling and intracellular events that collapse the cytoskeletal structure of basal keratinocytes with consequent shrinkage of these cells. Shrinking basal cells pull away from suprabasal cells, resulting in suprabasal acantholysis, and from each other, resulting in the "tombstone" appearance of basal cells. [314] The cytoskeleton of keratinocytes changes with retraction of intracellular keratin intermediate filaments from the cell periphery and clusters in a perinuclear position. [311] This is followed by breaking of the bond between tonofilaments and desmosomes, culminating in shrinkage of the basal cells. The detachment of tonofilaments occurs before the desmosomes show any visible alteration or loss in adhesion. [220] The final event in pemphigus vulgaris is acantholysis restricted to the basal cell layer. The keratinocyte cytoskeletal structure is affected to a greater extent by a signalling event and /or different set of signalling events is triggered in basal cells. The shrinkage hypothesis explained this event as follows: the binding of PV antibodies to keratinocytes causes changes in their cytoskeletal structure with consequent partial collapse and shrinkage of the cells. Keratinocytes separate because they shrink more than they can be held together by desmosomes, not because of a primary defect in the function of desmosomes; the shrinkage is limited to basal cells in pemphigus vulgaris because basal cells are less rigid and shrink more readily when their cytoskeleton is altered. [314]

Recently, one advanced study elucidated the molecular mechanism that selectively targets basal cells in pemphigus vulgaris, as predicted by the basal cell shrinkage hypothesis. Pretel et al. demonstrated that pretreatment with the mTOR[9] inhibitor sirolimus prevented suprabasal acantholysis in the epidermis of neonatal mice injected with PV antibodies. [296] The study observation supported that a restriction of acantholysis to the basal layer may be due, at least in part, to the selective and increased presence of activated HER[10] receptor isoforms in these cells. After phosphorylation of HER receptor isoforms, intracellular signalling pathways are activated in the basal layer. In this model, PV antibodies caused unopposed upregulation of mTOR selectively in basal keratinocytes, which was associated with the appearance of signs of apoptosis that were abolished by sirolimus. [296] Sirolimus has been shown to inhibit the expression of both c-Myc and Cdk2 that induces apoptosis. [315, 316] Taken together, these observations elucidated why epidermal acantholysis in pemphigus vulgaris always occurs just above basal cells, despite the deposition of PV antibodies throughout the entire epidermis.

Both extrinsic and intrinsic pathways of apoptosis triggered in keratinocytes by PV antibodies can lead to basal cell shrinkage. It has been documented *in vitro* that keratinocyte apoptosis precede their detachment and blister formation. Furthermore, PV antibodies and PV sera induce biomolecular markers of apoptosis and oncosis in keratinocyte monolayers and skin organ cultures. [317] Keratinocyte detachment and death in pemphigus vulgaris stem from the synergic action of the effectors of apoptosis and oncosis. It has been documented that PV antibodies from different patients proceed via separate pathways, namely apoptosis and oncosis, and that there exist two populations of patients, each producing PV antibodies that predominantly activate either a pro-apoptotic or pro-oncotic pathway of programmed cell death in keratinocytes. [317]

Apoptosis as a programmed cell death mechanism is characterized by a number of cytological and biochemical features as follows: nuclear condensation, activation of caspase cystein proteinases, DNA fragmentation, cell shrinkage, and membrane blebbing. [318] Apoptosis has been proposed to have a role in the mechanism by which PV antibodies induce keratinocyte death, followed by acantholysis. [319] The occurrence of apoptotic markers has been observed in early lesions of PV patients before acantholysis. TUNEL[11] positive keratinocytes indicating DNA fragmentation characteristic of cells undergoing apoptosis and other components of the pro-apoptotic pathway such as caspases, PERP or FAS have been

---

[9] mTOR (the mammalial target of rapamycin) signaling pathway integrates both intra- and extracellular signals and serves as a central regulator of cell metabolism, growth, proliferation and survival. This pathway is important in apoptosis. Deregulation is present in diseases such as cancer and type 2 diabetes. In many cancers it is overactive, thus reducing apoptosis and allowing proliferation.

[10] HER receptor isoforms are members of epidermal growth factor receptor family. Signalling through these receptors promotes cell proliferation, and opposes apoptosis. These receptors activate pathways including mitogen-activated protein kinase (MAPK), phosphoinositide 3-kinase (PI3K/Akt), protein kinase (PKC), signal transduce and activator of transcription (STAT) and phospholipase Cγ.

[11] TUNEL method detects DNA damage in situ. It is terminal deoxynucleotid transferase (TdT)- mediated dUTP-biotin nick end labeling staining. The method detects DNA fragmentation by labeling the terminal end of nucleic acids.

demonstrated in both lesional samples of pemphigus vulgaris and pemphigus foliaceus and in perilesional pemphigus skin. [319-322]

The anti-PERP IgG antibody in pemphigus vulgaris may initiate the cell death pathways in keratinocytes, because PERP expression leads to activation of an extrinsic receptor-mediated apoptotic pathway with possible subsequent insertion of the intrinsic apoptotic pathway. [323] In keratinocytes, the intrinsic apoptotic cascade can also be triggered by anti-mitochodrial IgG antibodies. [324] Several studies demonstrated other soluble mediators of inflammation that can activate the cell death pathway in keratinocytes. Upregulation of soluble Fas ligand in either PV sera and/or skin, suggesting that apoptosis in the skin is triggered via the Fas/FasL system. [319, 321, 325] Interestingly, anti-FasL blocking antibodies only partially inhibited this pro-apoptotic effect in PV sera on cultured keratinocytes, suggesting that other mechanism may contribute to inducing apoptosis.

Inflammatory cytokines TNF-α, IFN-γ and IL-1 were detected in the lesion exudates of pemphigus foliaceus patients, which may lead to the suggestion that inflammatory mediators could contribute to the induction of apoptosis in pemphigus. [322] Similarly, another study demonstrated that CD8+FasL+lymphocytes in pemphigus vulgaris skin may play a role in inducing apoptosis. [327] The PV antibody-depleted sera caused a sharp reduction of cell viability along with a less sustained weakening of intercellular adhesion strength.

Besides PV antibodies, cell death pathways in pemphigus can be triggered by autocrine and paracrine factors released from damaged keratinocytes *in situ*. The blister fluid and perilesional skin in pemphigus vulgaris patients contain high levels of various inflammatory cytokines and proteases that may contribute to acantholysis. [326, 327]

Taken together, acantholysis in pemphigus vulgaris occurs as a result of the cooperating action of both antibody and non-antibody mediated mechanisms. A simultaneous autoimmune attack could be mediated by antibodies directed against desmosomal autoantigens, other keratinocytes autoantigens, including mitochondrial, acetylcholine receptors and PERP that may be required to induce pathological changes leading to acantholysis. All these antibodies synergize with effectors of the apoptotic pathway FasL and TNFα and also with pro-inflammatory/cytotoxic serum and tissue factors such as serine proteases and cytokines.

In pemphigus, acantholysis and apoptosis/oncosis are inseparable and are triggered by the same signal effectors activated due to PV antibodies binding to keratinocytes and mediated by the same set of cell death enzymes. This is documented by the inhibition of Src, EGFRK, p38 MAPK, and mTOR that block both acantholysis and apoptosis. [296, 297, 327, 329-333] Furthermore, the cleavage of desmosomal proteins, namely Dsg1, Dsg2 and Dsg3, is orchestrated by caspases, leading to dissolution of cell structure and morphology. [334, 335] Additionally, anti-mitochondrial antibodies against various poorly defined mitochondrial autoantigens appear to have the ability to penetrate keratinocytes and react with mitochondrial proteins. The downstream signalling of anti-mitochondrial antibodies involves JNK and late p38 MAPK activation, thus underlying the important role for these signalling cascades in non-Dsg3 or non -Dsg1 autoantibody-specific autoimmune blistering. [163]

The structural damage and death of keratinocytes in pemphigus vulgaris are mediated by the same set of enzymes. The term apoptolysis differentiate the unique mechanism of autoantibody-induced keratinocyte damage in pemphigus vulgaris from another known form of cell death. [328] The classic apoptosis seen in toxic epidermal necrolysis (TEN) leads to cell death in epidermal layers and sloughing of the full thickness necrotic epidermis.

In difference, apoptosis in pemphigus vulgaris revealed basal cells shrink, rending a "tombstone" appearance to the basal layer. The fundamental difference between apoptolysis and apoptosis in pemphigus vulgaris is that the basal cells shrink but do not die. Grando et al. elaborated a novel apoptolysis concept that includes five consecutive steps:

1. The binding of autoantibodies to desmogleins, acetylcholine receptors and other members of the pemphigus antigen family on the plasma membrane of keratinocytes, sending an array of outside-in signals.
2. Activation of EGFR, Src, mTOR, p38MAPK and other signalling elements downstream of ligated antigens, elevation of intracellular Ca^{2+} and the launching of cell death cascades.
3. Early acantholysis manifested by basal cell shrinkage due to: collapse and retraction of the tonofilaments cleaved by executioner caspases; and dissociation of inter-desmosomal adhesion complexes caused by phosphorylation of adhesion molecules.
4. Massive cleavage of cellular proteins by activated cell death enzymes leading to cell collapse, and tearing off desmosomes from the cell membrane stimulating secondary autoantibody production.
5. Rounding up and death of acantholytic cells. Thus the structural damage (acantholysis) and death (apoptosis) of keratinocytes are mediated by the same cell death enzymes. [328] Figure 1.9. modified from ref. [328]

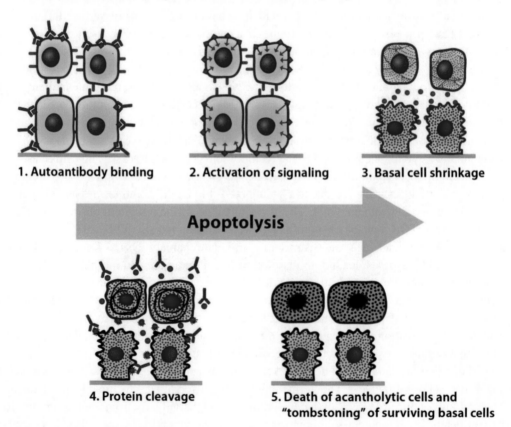

Figure 1.9. Hypothetical scheme of apoptolysis.

Apoptolysis is triggered by the binding of PV antibodies to various autoantigens capable of transducing apoptolytic signals from the keratinocyte plasma membrane. The collapse and retraction of tonofilaments and dissociation of inter-desmosomal adhesion complexes result in basal cell shrinkage, while most desmosomes remain intact. This is a crossing point of the apoptolytic lines and pemphigus acantholytic lines. The cleavage of cellular proteins leads to collapse of the cytoskeleton and the tearing off of desmosomes from the cell membrane, with subsequent production of scavenging autoantibodies, mainly to shed adhesion molecules. Suprabasal acantholytic cells die, allowing suprabasal blister formation and the constitution of "tombstone" basal cells. Scheme of apoptolysis modified from ref. [328]

Due to the diversity of self-antigens that have been reported to bind PV antibodies on the keratinocyte plasma membrane and reciprocal heterogeneity of anti-keratinocyte autoantibodies produced by individual patients, the signalling pathways elicited by PV antibodies from different patients are also expected to differ. Multiple adhesion molecules, as well as acetylcholine receptors and other keratinocyte proteins, have been referred to bind PV antibodies on the plasma membrane of keratinocytes and thus initiate receptor mobilization /aggregation and downstream signalling as described in the "multiple hit" hypothesis. [202] A recent discovery is discussed about the antigen specificity of the pathogenic antibodies initiating apoptolysis that the anti-Dsg antibodies, a diagnostic hallmark of pemphigus, may not always be pathogenic, instead playing the role of witness versus principal activator. [184] Keratinocytes shrink because the cytoskeleton collapses, presaging the beginning of acantholysis. Electron microscopy studies appointed that the shrinkage of basal cells associated with tonofilaments retraction is the earliest histopathological event in pemphigus vulgaris. [336, 337] In consonance with basal cell shrinkage hypothesis, the acantholysis occurs despite retention of desmosome adhesive properties, not because these properties are lost. [314] In successive steps that lead to acantholysis, proteolytic enzymes, such as caspases, cause collapse of the cytoskeleton with consequent collapse and shrinkage of the cells, whereas desmosomal separation occurs as the final and not as a primary or causative event of acantholysis. [310, 312] The desmosomal proteins Dsg3, Dsg1, plakoglobin, and desmoplakin as well as keratin intermediate filaments, have been demonstrated to undergo caspase-dependent cleavage. [338-340]. Furthermore, caspases may also regulate matrix metalloproteinase (MMP) dependent cleavage of desmogleins. [339]

Cell separation is released by dissolution of desmosomal adhesion complexes as well as adherens junction that facilitate cells to separate more easily as they collapse. Two sets of enzymes participated in the separation event. The first event includes cell death enzymes as caspases and calpain that have proteolytic activity. Caspases lead to cell death via apoptosis and calpain kills cells via oncosis. [341, 338] Both are induced by PV antibodies. [317] Tonofilaments are cleaved from their attachment to desmosomes and retract to the nucleus. The second event is phosphorylation of adhesion junction molecules executed by activated serine/threonine kinases. As a result, there is dissociation of adhesion complexes and their internalization for Dsg3, thus allowing shrinking cells to separate more easily. [288, 342, 343] It is suggested that the location of the epidermal split just above the basal cells may be caused by particularities of each signalling pathway and the molecular organization of the cytoskeleton. [296] Other studies supported these particularities by demonstrating certain types of keratin tonofilaments which can protect cell from apoptosis. [344, 345] In addition, PV sera have been shown to induce alterations in the cell cycle progression, which is unique to basal cells. [346] Acantholysis is spotty because only several basal cells are at the stage of active mitosis and therefore stigmatized with PV antibodies, which subsequently induce shrinkage of the basal cells. [328]

In conclusion, the exclusive role of anti-Dsg1 and Dsg3 antibodies in pemphigus vulgaris pathogenesis, which causes steric hindrance at the adhesion points of keratinocytes, has been largely reevaluated. The pathologic outcome of PV antibody-induced signalling is induction of the apoptotic and/or oncotic pathways, associated with the collapse of the cytoskeleton. The outside-in signalling of PV antibody can be evoked through cholinergic receptors and desmosomal proteins, as well as other yet unknown antigen or receptors ligated on the cell membrane of keratinocyte as explicated by the "multiple -hit "hypothesis. The major downstream signalling event is considered to result from activation of acetylcholine receptors expressed in keratinocytes. The outside-in signalling elicited due to the binding of PV antibodies to keratinocytes proceeds via different pathways, consistent with simultaneous ligation of several types of cell surface receptors by distinct antibodies produced by pemphigus patients. The binding of PV antibody triggers signalling and intracellular events that collapse the cytoskeletal structure of basal keratinocytes with consequent shrinkage of these cells. The final event in pemphigus vulgaris is acantholysis restricted to the basal cell layer. It is supposed, that a simultaneous autoimmune attack could be mediated by antibodies directed against desmosomal autoantigens, other keratinocytes autoantigens, including mitochondrial, acetylcholine receptors and PERP that may be required to induce pathological changes leading to acantholysis.

Triggers in Pemphigus Vulgaris

During the past 20 years, a significant increase has been observed in the incidence of autoimmune disease worldwide. The observation is targeted to the etiology and pathogenesis of autoimmune diseases, including pemphigus vulgaris. It does appear that a close interplay between exogenous triggers and genetic factors is responsible for the loss of immunological tolerance and autoimmunity. Therefore, in relation to the role of heritability in autoimmune disease, genome-wide association studies reported that genetics only accounted for a minority of cases with autoimmune disease. For this reason, research and publications dedicated to exogenous factors in autoimmune diseases. Generally, this includes toxic chemicals, infections and dietary components. Overall, the precise mechanism of exogenously induced autoimmune disease is unknown. Recently, it was documented that exogenous triggers can induce changes in gene expression. For example, environmental pollutants, cigarette smoke and alcohol consumption have been advocated for increased incidence in autoimmune diseases due to their links with the induction of DNA methylation. [347] Toxicants, infections, dysfunctions of immune homeostasis, and dietary components, can all have an impact on the human immune recognition system. Although the precise etiology and pathogenesis of many autoimmune diseases are still unknown, it would appear from collated studies that there are common conformable mechanisms in the immunopathogenesis of multiple autoimmune diseases.

In genetically predisposed individuals, exogenous triggers can induce the formation of neoantigens, or be capable of inducing the citrullination[12] of host proteins and converting them to autoantigens. Thus, these modified proteins can be recognized by the immune system, and subsequently can trigger antibody production and the inflammatory process involved in the clinical manifestation of autoimmune diseases. [348] Thus, several exogenous factors have been implicated.

In pemphigus vulgaris, the genetic predisposition is known to be associated with declaratory HLA loci. Two HLA class II subtypes, DRB1*0402 and DQB1*0503, have been mostly linked to the disease. Accordingly, over 95% of patients carry at least one of these alleles. [46] As stated in previous subchapter, it should be noted that the majority of genetically, predisposed individuals do not develop disease. [180, 190, 192] The genetic background alone, though essential, is not by itself sufficient to induce the autoimmune response. The intervention of inducing or triggering factors seems to be crucial to activate the full-blown disease. Several exogenous factors may induce processes in the skin that promote the exposure of self-antigens and the development of subsequent and progressive humoral autoimmunity. Exogenous factors may cause immune dysregulation, leading to autoimmunity, or autoimmunity by molecular mimicry. Factors causing keratinocyte necrosis propose a potential mechanism for release of intracellular molecules, which are then exposed to autoreactive T cells. Induced inflammatory or autoimmune disease process can cause tissue damage and introduce certain protein tissue components originally hidden from autoreactive T cells or B cells. This exposure evokes a primary or secondary autoimmune response. [349] Despite this, in the majority of patients, no trigger factor can be detected and the disease apparently starts in a spontaneous manner (termed spontaneous or idiopathic pemphigus vulgaris). In other cases, a precise clinical history discloses trigger factors (termed induced or triggered pemphigus vulgaris). In induced pemphigus vulgaris the exogenous factors play a major role, so that the condition regresses after the inducing factor has been eliminated, even in the absence of any treatment. The most frequent variant is drug-induced pemphigus, usually differing from spontaneous pemphigus vulgaris for clinical features. Induced pemphigus conditions mostly resemble pemphigus foliaceus or pemphigus herpetiformis; histology reveals an acantholysis being irregular and not neatly suprabasilar. Triggered pemphigus vulgaris refers to a condition where endogenous factors are more important and the trigger factors only induce a disease, in a causal and non-specific manner. Despite the elimination of the trigger factor, the disease self-perpetuates with all characteristics of spontaneous pemphigus, in particular of pemphigus vulgaris. [350]

Exogenous factors that may induce or trigger pemphigus vulgaris are numerous and heterogeneous, encompassing several drugs e.g., anti-rheumatic and NSAIDs, antibiotics, chemotherapies, antihypertensive drugs, cytokines, and others. Other triggers embrace some viral infections (e.g., herpes virus), physical agents (e.g., thermal burns, ultraviolet and ionizing radiation), including surgical and cosmetic procedures, and contact allergens (e.g., pesticides). However, endogenous factors and even emotional stress being related to the individual lifestyle may trigger or aggravate disease. In the majority of patients with pemphigus vulgaris, any trigger factor is obvious and the disease seems to start in a

---

[12] Protein citrullination means the changing of an amino acid from arginine to citrulline. This can result in immune reaction against the original protein or its citrullinated form, additionally also against other citrullinated proteins.

spontaneous manner. However, in several cases the presence of trigger factors that can lead to the onset of pemphigus vulgaris is often suspected on the basis of circumstantial evidence, but sometimes it can be demonstrated without evidence.

A large series of medications can induce or trigger pemphigus vulgaris. A precise history taking is needed to determine the culprit medication. Such a history should include any kinds of drugs, including over-the-counter drugs. The causal relationship between drug and disease has been generally based on a temporal correlation in both outbreak and remission, rather than on *in vitro* confirmation as a re-challenge in pemphigus vulgaris is not a medical option. The mechanism of drug-induced pemphigus is still obscure.

There are three groups of chemicals that may induce pemphigus as follows: sulfhydryl radical (thiol drugs or SH drugs); phenol drugs; and nonthiol nonphenol drugs. Thiol drugs containing or releasing a sulfhydryl radical include penicillamine, bucillamine, captopril and gold sodium thiomalate. Rifampin, levodopa, cephadroxil, cefoperazone, phenobarbital, aspirin and heroin are examples of phenol drugs. Heroin and aspirin are "masked phenols" in the sense that they induce phenols following metabolism. Nonthiol nonphenol drugs include nonsteroidal anti-inflammatory drugs (NSAIDs), angiotensin-converting enzyme (ACE) inhibitors, calcium channel blockers, glibenclamide, and dipyrone. Furthermore, some drugs assess both thiol and phenol ring components and thus can promote pemphigus by two different pathways (e.g., some cephalosporins, pyritinol and 5-thiopyridoxine). Drugs implicated in the induction of pemphigus are grouped according to their chemical structure. Table 1.1. modified from ref [351]

Table 1.1. Drugs involved in triggering pemphigus vulgaris according to their chemical structure

Thiols (sulphydryl radicals)	Phenols
Penicillamine	Aspirin
Bucillamine	Cephalosporins *
Penicillin	Rifampin
Thiopronine	Levodopa
Gold sodium thiomalate	Heroin
Piroxicam	Pentachlorophenol
Captopril	Phenobarbital
Pyaritinol	**Non-thiol non-phenol drugs**
5-thiopyridoxine	ACE-inhibitors other than captopril
Thiamazole	Most NSAID
Nifedipine	Nifedipine
Vaccines, interferons, cytokines	Vaccines, interferons, cytokines
Others	Others

Legend: ACE, angiotensin-converting enzyme; NSAID, nosteroidal anti-inflammatory drug.
    *Some cephalosporines are both thiol and phenol drugs.

The first drug reported to induce pemphigus was D-penicillamine, the prototype of thiol drugs. Experimental studies have demonstrated that thiol drugs were capable of inducing acantholysis directly in human skin explants in the absence of autoantibody, probably by direct toxic effect via direct binding with keratinocytes and drugs. [352] The expected mechanisms for acantholysis induced by thiol drugs embrace the inhibition of enzymes that aggregate keratinocytes and activation of enzymes that disaggregate keratinocytes, leading to the formation of thiol-cysteine instead of cysteine-cysteine bonds resulting in cell-cell adhesion disturbance. This phenomenon has been termed biochemical acantholysis, which led to a non-antibody-mediated pemphigus-like syndrome. On the other hand, thiol drugs can lead to alterations of the antigenic structure of desmogleins binding with drugs through a thiol-disulfide interchange, thereby cleaving the PV antigen or rendering it nonfunctional. In addition, alteration of the desmoglein molecule is followed by binding of the drug with consequent formation of a neoantigen eliciting an immune response resulting in the production of anti-Dsg antibodies. [353] In thiol drugs-induced pemphigus, the prevalence of PV antibodies is lower than that in spontaneously occurring pemphigus. [354, 355] Thiol drugs have either a sulfhydryl (-SH) group in their structure, such as penicillamine and captopril, or contain a disulfide bond releasing SH groups, such as gold and pyritiol. The clinical appearance of thiol drug-induced pemphigus is usually pemphigus foliaceus, potentially due to the existence of many SH groups at the spino-granular junction in the epidermis. [356, 357]. In addition, rare cases of pemphigus vulgaris induced by bucillamine, structurally similar to penicillamine, were documented in literature. [353, 354] The thiol drugs have more frequently been involved in triggered pemphigus vulgaris, including penicillamine, captopril, and penicillin and its derivatives (mainly aminopenicillins), piroxicam, gold sodiumthiomalate and thiamazole. [351, 358] It should be mentioned that gold sodium thiomalate is a contradictory drug because it can facilitate the onset of pemphigus vulgaris. On the other hand, it can be used in the treatment of pemphigus vulgaris as an alternative therapy.

A possible mechanism for phenol-induced pemphigus vulgaris in genetically predisposed individuals is proposed that the drug may induce the release of cytokines such as TNFα, IL-1 and IL-8 from keratinocytes. [359] These cytokines have been shown to be implicated in the pathogenesis of acantholysis. [360] Cephalosporins (mainly the injectable ones, e.g., ceftriaxone) and aspirin are the most frequently used phenol drugs responsible for inducing pemphigus vulgaris in genetically predisposed individuals. In addition, topical phenol was referred to induce pemphigus vulgaris in genetically susceptible patients. [361]

Calcium channel blockers may induce pemphigus vulgaris by the pathway of a decreased level of Ca^{2+}, because desmogleins are calcium -dependent and additionally enzymes possessing keratinization are also calcium-dependent. [362] Furthermore, drugs with the active amide group, and quinolone can be capable of inducing pemphigus vulgaris in genetically predisposed individuals. [363, 364] In both drugs, the mechanism how they can induce pemphigus vulgaris is still unknown. Among drugs capable of facilitating the outbreak of pemphigus vulgaris are also the biologic modifiers of the immune response, such as vaccines, interferons and other cytokines that may promote acantholysis. [351]

Two decades ago, up to 10% of cases of pemphigus in Western countries were drug-induced, with the disease beginning weeks or months after initial drug exposure. [365] The drugs involved in the induction of pemphigus were mainly penicillamine and more rarely, other drugs containing a thiol radical, namely piroxicam, captopril or other ACE inhibitors. With limitation penicillamine use, the incidence of drug-induced pemphigus was reduced.

An immune disease can be induced or triggered by infectious agents. Most infectious agents such as viruses, bacteria, fungi, and parasites can induce autoimmunity via different mechanisms. In many cases, it is not a single infection but rather the "burden of infections" from childhood that is responsible for the induction of autoimmunity. The development of an autoimmune disease after infection tends to occur in genetically predisposed individuals. [366] During the past 50 years, molecular techniques have been used to investigate the interaction between infections and autoimmunity. [348] A large number of viruses have been associated with a variety of autoimmune conditions, but an absolute link has not been established. A trigger mechanism is proposed: viruses can stimulate the immune response in genetically predisposed individuals leading to an increase in the production of IFNγ and cytokines. After that, high levels of IFNγ can induce the expression of molecules HLA class II, making the structural site of desmosomal cadherins immunologically active and inducing epitope spreading. Infectious agents such as viruses and bacteria were reported as preceding or exacerbating pemphigus disease. In addition, chronic viral infection has been found to promote a shift from Th1 to Th2, with the up-regulation of IL-4 and IL-10, supporting humoral response. [348] Several viruses have been blamed for triggering or exacerbating pemphigus disease. Numerous studies documented that the prevalence of antibodies directed at various viruses including herpes simplex virus, hepatitis B virus, hepatitis C virus, toxoplasmosis and cytomegalovirus, were significantly higher in patients with pemphigus vulgaris compared with controls. [367]. Recently, it was referred that patients with pemphigus vulgaris have also a significantly higher prevalence of antibodies against *Helicobacter pylori, Toxoplasma gondii* in comparison to controls. [368] These results allow speculation about the contributing role for the mentioned microbial and parasitic agents in the pathogenesis of pemphigus vulgaris. Perhaps the most studied group of viral pathogens is that of herpes viruses, with considerable evidence linking *the herpes simplex virus* (HSV) and pemphigus vulgaris. HSVs have been referred to influence the course of the disease and have been associated with pemphigus vulgaris flares and clinical exacerbations, or can simply complicate its clinical course. Furthermore, HSV infection can induce the production of autoantibodies through molecular mimicry originating from epithelial tissue damage by HSV. However, the presence of HSV in perpetuating PV lesions cannot be excluded because of iatrogenic immunosuppression from corticosteroids and other immunosuppressant used in the treatment of patients with pemphigus vulgaris, and on the other hand from the lack of normal epithelial barrier in PV lesions. However, it has been documented that HSV infection is not accompanied by an increase in anti-Dsg antibodies. [369] Taken together, HSV infection may only be an occasional trigger factor that can induce the outbreak or exacerbation of pemphigus vulgaris through a nonspecific way. The same ascertainment could be held for other common viral infections, including flu, cold, and other infections of the upper respiratory tract. In addition, a concurrent facilitating effect might be due to the use of drugs such as penicillin derivates, cephalosporins, pyrazolones, and other NSAIDs usually employed in the management of viral infections to prevent bacterial super-infections and being suspected of inducing pemphigus vulgaris.

On the other hand, some studies demonstrated detection of HSV in the lesions of patients during multiple flares of pemphigus vulgaris. However, the detection of HSV infection that occurs during clinical flares did not correlate with an increase in anti-Dsg3 antibodies. [369] Generally, the lack of demonstration of consistent HSV infection in PV patients seems to suggest that HSV infection may exacerbate or prolong the PV lesions rather than participate as a primary cause of the disease. Patients with recalcitrant PV lesions are more likely to be infected with HSV, whereas those without recalcitrant PV lesions are likely to be negative for HSV infection. [370] Healing of the PV lesions after acyclovir therapy suggests that HSV infection may play a role in exacerbation, even if it is not directly causative. [371, 372] One can suggest that the HSV infection in patients with pemphigus vulgaris leads to a worsening of the disease's symptoms by affecting cellular and humoral factors of immunity, which ultimately exacerbate or worsen PV lesions. On the other hand, it may be possible that HSV is a secondary infection in patients with pemphigus vulgaris taking immunosuppressive therapy, which render their immune system vulnerable to viral attack. Recently, in one study, high levels of HSV DNA in the saliva samples were discovered at the earlier stage of pemphigus vulgaris. The level of HSV DNA was transient and later became undetectable when anti-HSV antibody titres increased, or alternatively when anti-Dsg antibody increased. [373] These results suggest that the HSV might have contributed to the initial phase of pemphigus vulgaris and then disappear once antiviral and autoimmune responses become fully established. Another study supported that HSV infection can reactivate or exacerbate persistent PV lesions and may complicate pemphigus vulgaris. [374, 375]

In addition, numerous studies evaluated the connection between various viruses including human herpes virus 8 (HHV-8), Ebstein Barr virus, cytomegalovirus and varicella-zoster virus, and their observations revealed contrary results. [376-380] The detection of viral antibodies or DNA has provided evidence for a potential role for viral agents in pemphigus vulgaris. Furthermore, several case reports documented that some viral infection preceded the development of pemphigus vulgaris, e.g., H1N1infection (swine flu), and varicella infection. [381, 382] Contrary reports have not found an association between inducing pemphigus vulgaris and hepatitis C and hepatitis B virus infections. [383] However, no clear association has been established between viral infection and pemphigus vulgaris, but viruses cannot be overlooked as possible trigger or exacerbating factors in pemphigus vulgaris.

Taken together, it has to be noted that currently no infectious agent has been confirmed as a causative trigger factor in pemphigus vulgaris. However, as with many autoimmune diseases, certain exogenous factors, such as herpes viruses, have been associated with disease onset and exacerbation and therefore viral infection cannot be ruled out from autoimmunity, the course and the outcome of autoimmune diseases, including pemphigus vulgaris.

Bacterial infections were not reported as an inducing factor in pemphigus. On the other hand, septicemia of *Staphylococcus aureus, Proteus vulgaris, Pseudomonas aeruginosa* and other microorganisms occurs as a complication of immunosuppressive therapy and not as a trigger that can induce pemphigus vulgaris. [384] Opportunistic infections were referred as a significant risk in the first year after PV diagnosis with potential deleterious effects. Infectious agents included *Nocardia, cytomegalovirus, Legionella*, and *Listeria*. [385] However, in staphylococcal scaled skin syndrome (SSSS), *Staphylococcus aureus* may produce exfoliate toxin A which especially binds to Dsg1 and causes a loss of cell-to-cell adhesion in the superficial epidermis similar to pemphigus foliaceus. [386, 387]

The induction of pemphigus vulgaris in genetically predisposed individuals by physical agents such as ultraviolet or ionizing radiation, thermal or electrical burns, surgery and cosmetic procedures, is documented in several reports.

Ultraviolet (UV) radiation is known to induce or aggravate several autoimmune diseases, including pemphigus vulgaris. The precise mechanism by which UV radiation is capable of triggering pemphigus vulgaris is not well understood, but several possible mechanisms have been proposed. UV and ionizing radiation can alter the biochemistry of the epidermis and on the other hand the regulatory mechanisms of autoimmunity. One proposed mechanism is that of the promotion of activation of intracellular signaling pathways after the binding of PV antibodies, and increased production of pro-inflammatory cytokines such as IL-1, TNFα and others. [103] UV radiation is considered to be the most important physical factor in induced pemphigus vulgaris. UV radiation has been documented to induce a transient form of pemphigus *de novo* in apparently healthy individuals; in others it exacerbates pre-existing pemphigus vulgaris. [388, 389]. In concordance with UV radiation induced pemphigus it was referred pemphigus vulgaris induced with PUVA therapy; it is suggested that UVA could be responsible for the inducing effect of sunlight exposure. [390, 391]

Ionizing radiation may induce or exacerbate various types of pemphigus, including pemphigus vulgaris, pemphigus foliaceus, and paraneoplastic pemphigus. [392-394] Most frequently, in ionizing radiation-induced pemphigus, a typical accentuation of the disease is developed in therapeutic radiation portal. [395] In general, the time interval between completion of irradiation and the appearance of the blister formation spanned between a few days up to 1 year. [396] However, an initial eruption appears during or after radiotherapy that is consistent with acute radiodermatitis, then there is a period of weeks before the onset of an initial eruption of disease within the radiation portal. [397]

Another physical agent that is capable of inducing pemphigus vulgaris is thermal or electrical burns. PV lesions appear within and adjacent to the burned areas and subsequently extend to other skin regions. [398, 399] The mechanism of thermal and electrical injury may cause protein denaturation and ultimately results in the destruction of tissue with the release of their cellular constituents. The operating mechanism may release desmogleins, pro-inflammatory mediators, and possibly cryptic peptides launching an inflammatory response. [398] These provocation physical stimuli can induce, in genetically predisposed individuals to pemphigus vulgaris, the specific antibody production responsible for immune-mediated acantholysis.

In literature, several cases referred that pemphigus vulgaris in genetically susceptible individuals can be induced by some chemicals such as chromium sulfate (used as occupational contact), and dihydrodiphenyltrichlorethane (used as pesticide). [400, 401] Another phenol compound, pentachlorophenol, is used as an insecticide, herbicide, fungicide and wood preservative. Pentachlorophenol is readily absorbed through the skin and can induce pemphigus vulgaris in genetically predisposed individuals. [402, 403] Another chemical is organophosphate pesticide, a cholinesterase inhibitor that causes an accumulation of acetylcholine at cholinergic receptors and could favor the development of acantholysis. [350] Furthermore, cosmetic procedures can induce pemphigus vulgaris as discussed in the literature. Topical phenol used as chemical peeling induced pemphigus vulgaris, and surgical procedures such as a reduction mammoplasty and facelift were responsible for induced pemphigus vulgaris in genetically predisposed individuals. [404] The mechanism of contact pemphigus vulgaris is considered to be a combination of direct alteration of the skin structure, with the possible activation of the immune system of the compound itself.

Nutritional compounds are rarely mentioned as possible triggers of pemphigus vulgaris. However, some nutritional components are biochemically similar to a causative drug that may induce pemphigus. The large amounts of thiols, phenols, and polyphenolic compounds like tannins led several authors to postulate that these foodstuffs may also induce and promote pemphigus vulgaris. The genus *Allium* of vegetables, which includes garlic, leeks and onion, are among the suspected foodstuffs. [405] These plants are rich in thiol allyl compounds with *in vitro* proven acantholytic potential. [406] Also tannins, polyphenolic compounds, contained in several plants and fruits and their derivates, e.g., black pepper, red chili pepper, cherry cranberry, blackberry, mango, avocado and red wine, have been considered to be capable of inducing pemphigus vulgaris in genetically predisposed individuals. Tannin is the main component of tea, manufactured and used in India. Experimentally, subjects with a diet rich in tannins had increased tannin metabolites in the suction blister and tannin showed acantholytic activity *in vitro.* [407] It is believed that tannin substances may either be incorporated into the epithelia, leading to biochemical acantholysis, or may release sequestered antigens and also interfere with the immune balance, leading to antibody-mediated immunological acantholysis. [408] Other plants and fruit may contain compounds like urushiol (3´5´-pentadecylcatechol) that are chemically similar with long-chain phenols that are suspected of inducing pemphigus. [409] Other suspected foods are those containing isothiocyanates such as mustard and horseradish. In addition, food can also contain phenols. One type of phenol is a cinnamic acid that can be found in fruit juice and flavorings used in the nutrition industry, e.g., ice cream. Another common type of phenol is a pinene found in potatoes and black pepper. Several foodstuffs may be active in inducing pemphigus vulgaris or pemphigus foliaceus in a geographic area with nutritional habituations of these nutritional products. The same chemical compound such as thiol or phenol in drugs may contain some foodstuff used habitually in certain geographic areas. The pathomechanisms could be both antibody -mediated acantholysis or biochemical acantholysis in a similar manner to thiol or phenol bearing drugs.

The etiology of the loss of normal self-tolerance in an autoimmune disease is multifactorial. Many studies had found that a high proportion (up to 80%) of patients reported uncommon psychological stress before disease onset. [ref.in 410] Stress itself is not considered to be an illness, but rather a state and long term stress may cause a serious health problem. The role of stress in the pathogenesis of autoimmune disease is controversial and not currently accepted as an etiologic factor. [410] However, stress affects the immune system and different stress reactions should be discussed with autoimmune patients including patients with pemphigus vulgaris. In addition, several cases of pemphigus vulgaris triggered by emotional stress have been reported. [411] Immunosuppressive treatment should be associated with psychological care, entailing better management of these patients. The stressing events have been lived in a highly emotional way such as war, terrorism, near relative´s death, separation from partner, sexual aggression or sex-related disturbance.

In literature, there are some reports about the influence of nicotine to the pemphigus. Some case reports demonstrated an improvement of pemphigus vulgaris by cigarette smoking. [349, 412] It could be explained by the acetylcholine network in the human oral mucosa. Especially, human keratinocytes synthesize, store, release and degrade acetylcholine. Both nicotinic and muscarinic acetylcholine receptors on the surface of keratinocytes regulate cell-to-cell adhesion. [160] It is speculated that interaction of nicotine with nicotinic acetylcholine receptors on keratinocytes may open ion gates in the cell membrane to help increase cell-to-cell adherence and to clear down acantholysis. [413] The protective effect of nicotine in pemphigus should encourage further investigations aimed at discovering novel therapies. However, it should be recommended not to forget the association of smoking with lung carcinoma and cardiac and peripheral vascular disease, as well as impaired wound healing.

In addition, according to several reports the most reported triggers for developing pemphigus vulgaris are emotional stress, medication, surgical or dental procedures, physical stress or trauma, and illness. Other factors associated with increased risk of initiation or exacerbation of pemphigus vulgaris are pesticides, metal vapors, and UV exposure. However, only 5.7% of the patients from an internet -based patients survey from the USA reported environmental triggers such as exposure to chemicals, toxins, or UV sun exposure. [10] In addition, influenza tetanus and diphtheria, hepatitis B, and antirabies vaccines have been previously suggested as trigger factors. [414-417] However, in the USA large internet-based study, only 2 patients recorded that vaccination against poliomyelitis or influenza led to the onset of pemphigus vulgaris. [10]

In conclusion, unlike hereditary and genetic factors cannot be changed; many lifestyle and environmental factors can be modified in order to better manage pemphigus disease.

PREDICTORS OF COURSE AND PROGNOSIS IN PEMPHIGUS VULGARIS

Pemphigus vulgaris typically has a chronic course with strong variability in terms of disease duration and the time taken to achieve disease remission among afflicted patients. Several authors tried to identify factors that may influence the prognosis of pemphigus vulgaris. In various studies many parameters were evaluated. Certain genetic, epidemiological, clinical and immunological factors may influence the prognosis of pemphigus vulgaris. It seems that especially the age of onset, initial severity and matching dose of initial corticosteroid treatment, duration of remission, rate of relapses, therapy complications and mortality, could be considered to have some prognostic value.

One of the predictors of the course of prognosis seems to be a phenotype of pemphigus vulgaris. Several clinical studies evaluated that the mucocutaneous phenotype is more frequent than the mucous phenotype and is considered to be more severe in occurrence. One study observed that patients with the mucocutaneous phenotype achieved later clinical control of the disease and they had a lower rate of remission at the end of the first and second years of treatment than those of the mucous or cutaneous phenotypes. [418] After the second year of treatment, 67% (59/88) of patients with mucocutaneous type had active disease compared with those of mucous or cutaneous phenotypes, 55.6% (20/36). [418]

The prognostic importance of mucosal involvement at the onset of disease is difficult to evaluate because of its high frequency in pemphigus vulgaris. Despite this, it was clearly demonstrated that involvement of oral mucosa at onset of the disease was strongly associated with poorer prognosis. [19] Another study supported mucosal involvement at presentation as a prognostic factor of poor outcome since it was significantly associated with a high rate of relapses (54.2% vs.17.4%) (p=0.015) and shorter first relapse-free survival time (1.28 vs. 3 years) (p=0.0017). [24] Furthermore, another study supported the mucosal involvement to impact the poor outcome of the disease. Mucosal involvement at onset of disease revealed a longer remission survival compared to those who had no initial mucosal changes (5years vs. 3.5 years). [33]

Another study evaluated initial first disease remission and the time taken to total disease duration. The authors found a positive correlation between both first disease remission and total disease duration, suggesting that if it is difficult to achieve initial control (disease remission), patients are more likely to have a longer overall disease duration. [419] In addition, differences in remission survival were also documented between patients with mild, moderate and severe pemphigus vulgaris (2.5 years vs. 4 years vs. 5 years). These results were supported by significant differences found in the number of relapses and initial disease severity (p=0.01). [33]

In literature, it was documented that ethnic group may influence the prognosis and outcome of pemphigus vulgaris. Indo-Asian patients had substantially longer disease duration than Caucasian European patients. [419] Only 3/35 (9%) Indo-Asian compared with 15/42 (36%) of Caucasian Europeans, had duration disease <5 years (p=0.016). Ethnic group differences are considered to be a prognostic factor also in other studies. Pemphigus vulgaris in Indian patients has been associated with the presence of both anti-Dsg 1 and anti-Dsg3 antibodies, leading to a more severe clinical phenotype. [420] These results are in concordance with another study that documented a correlation of the initial high level of anti-Dsg3 antibody and a poorer prognosis of pemphigus vulgaris. [421] Also initial intercellular antibody titre on human skin substrate was associated with a greater time to initial disease remission and high anti-Dsg3 antibody levels with longer disease duration. [419]

Other reports documented inconsistent data about the relevance age at disease onset. A young age at disease onset was identified to be a significant independent predictor of poor outcome of pemphigus vulgaris in the Jewish population when compared with the onset of disease between younger individuals under 40 years of age and older ones. [19] On the other hand, another study found no influence of age in terms of disease control and in terms of the first relapse-free survival time, when they compared young adults under 40 and patients aged 40 years and more. [24] A recent study supported the last results and documented no influence of age on remission survival. [33] Whereas, by comparing patients under 65 years old and elderly patients, the healing time was significantly longer in adults under 65, but there was no difference in terms of the first relapse-free survival time between these two age groups. [24] These results were supported by another study, where age at onset did not reveal longer disease duration or time of initial first disease remission. However, in the group of patients who have had the disease duration time <5 years, age at presentation was associated with slightly older patients (49 years SEM 3.4 compared with 40years SEM 1.9) (p=0.039). [419]

Furthermore, it was observed that remission survival was significantly longer in females than in males (5 years vs. 3 years) (p=0.003). [33] This finding is consistent with other results in the study. Women suffered from severe pemphigus vulgaris more frequently than men (female: male ratio: 2.8), more frequently they had multiple mucosal involvement and were younger at the onset of disease. These results contrast with those of recent studies that did not observe gender-based differences, although other authors have reported a young age at disease onset (<40 years) and primary mucosal involvement to be associated with a poor prognosis. [19]

The genetic impact to the prognosis and outcome of pemphigus vulgaris was recently investigated. Dhandha et al. documented that carriers of one or both HLA DRB1 *04:02 and DQB1*05:03 produce significantly higher levels of anti -Dsg3 antibody than carriers of other HLA alleles. [111] In addition, Svecova et al. documented that patients carrying HLA DRB1*04:02 far more frequently revealed severe pemphigus vulgaris and more frequently have the mucocutaneous phenotype than those carrying other HLA alleles. Moreover, the study documented an association of HLA DQB1*03:02 in patients with severe pemphigus vulgaris and in female patients. [15] These results were in concordance with the author's previous study, in which they documented more severe levels of the disease in female than in male patients with pemphigus vulgaris. [33] To the best our knowledge, these two studies provided the first evidence supporting how HLA antigens impact the severity of pemphigus disease and influence the prognosis of the disease.

All environmental factors may alter the immune response and further impact the prognosis of pemphigus vulgaris, as mentioned in previous subchapter. In addition, the role of acetylcholine receptors, both nicotinic and muscarinic, plays an essential role in stimulating keratinocytes to maintain their shape and connection to each other. Nicotine is considered to be a direct acting cholinergic agonist and may be interfering with the activity of anti-acetylcholine receptors antibodies in pemphigus vulgaris. A few clinical studies have confirmed the beneficial effect of cholinergic agonist, such as nicotine and pilocarpine gel, in the treatment of pemphigus. [422, 423] Based on this theory, nicotine may improve keratinocyte adhesion functions. Several studies showed the positive impact of nicotine in smokers to the development of pemphigus. One study documented a decreased risk of pemphigus in former or current smokers, compared with controls. [258] Another study referred that smoking did not affect the rate of cutaneous or mucosal involvement in pemphigus; however remission has been achieved sooner in patients who smoke. [424] The recent study found that the rate of smokers in the population and pemphigus patients significantly did not differ and so the influence to disease duration or disease remission could not be evaluated. [419] According to these results, the role of nicotine abuse in the prognosis of pemphigus needs more cohorts, especially in populations with more habitual smoking.

In conclusion, despite pemphigus vulgaris having an unpredictable course, there are several studies that evaluated the association of certain clinical, epidemiological, immunological and genetic parameters that may influence the course and prognosis of disease. Pemphigus is a rare disease and to find a correlation between various aspects implicated in the pathogenesis of the disease requires a large number of patients and this fact complicates the evaluation of previous and also future studies.

CONCLUSION

Pemphigus vulgaris is very rare disease and the epidemiology varies across the world. The numerous studies documented that pemphigus vulgaris is the most frequent condition inside the pemphigus disease group, especially in Europe and North America. The highest incidence is documented in several populations, including the Jewish population, in particular of Ashkenazi origin, in individuals of Mediterranean descent and in the Japanese and Indian populations. It seems that the Romany population may also belong to this entity. In general, autoimmune diseases are more frequent in female. In concordance with this many epidemiological studies revealed a female preponderance. The prevalence of other autoimmune diseases is high in patients with pemphigus vulgaris, mostly of thyroid gland. Autoimmune comorbidity is also frequent in relatives; however, they do not suffer from pemphigus vulgaris.

Genetic background of pemphigus vulgaris was confirmed in numerous studies. Among alleles positively associated in Caucasian patients with pemphigus vulgaris belong HLA DRB1*04:02, DRB1*14:01, DRB1*14:04 and HLA DQB1*05:03 and DQB1*03:02. Recently, a new allele HLA DRB1*14:54 was discovered in association with pemphigus vulgaris, so far documented only in two studies. In the meantime, this allele was included in

DRB1*14:01 because they both differ in a single sole nucleotide. By reevaluating the pemphigus vulgaris population from various destinations, the account of HLA DRB1*14:54 should be probably enhanced. The strong genetic background in patients with pemphigus vulgaris was confirmed by evidence of HLA haplotypes associated with pemphigus vulgaris that are present in 95% of PV patients.

The exclusive role of anti-Dsg1 and Dsg3 antibodies in pemphigus vulgaris pathogenesis, which causes steric hindrance at the adhesion points of keratinocytes, has been largely reevaluated. The pathologic outcome of PV antibody-induced signalling is induction of the apoptotic and/or oncotic pathways, associated with the collapse of the cytoskeleton. The outside-in signalling of PV antibody can be evoked through cholinergic receptors and desmosomal proteins, as well as other yet unknown antigen or receptors ligated on the cell membrane of keratinocyte as explicated by the "multiplehit "hypothesis. The major downstream signalling event is considered to result from activation of cholinergic receptors expressed in keratinocytes. The binding of PV antibody triggers signalling and intracellular events that collapse the cytoskeletal structure of basal keratinocytes with consequent shrinkage of these cells. The final event in pemphigus vulgaris is acantholysis restricted to the basal cell layer. According to these findings anti-Dsg3 and anti-Dsg1antibody loosed their priority in PV autoimmunity. However, their position remains important because they possess the induction of autoantibodies that correlate with the clinical activity of the disease.

Research of autoimmunity dysregulation in pemphigus vulgaris discovered molecules known also in pathogenesis of other autoimmune disorders such as Th17 cells, Treg and Breg. Interestingly, Treg cells are required for maintenance of peripheral tolerance and homeostasis and are higher in healthy individuals with HLA class II alleles associated with pemphigus vulgaris than in patients with active pemphigus vulgaris. A decrease in Treg cells in peripheral blood of patients with pemphigus vulgaris does not validate the postulated deficiency of the immunosuppressive activity, because Treg cells are present in PV lesions. The role of other regulatory cells such as Breg cells in the autoimmunity of pemphigus vulgaris remains to be determined, as well as the putative interplay between Treg cells and Th17 cells.

Despite pemphigus vulgaris having an unpredictable course, there are several studies evaluated the association of certain clinical, epidemiological, immunological and genetic parameters that may predict the course of prognosis of disease. One such a predictor seems to be a phenotype of pemphigus vulgaris. Several clinical studies evaluated that the mucocutaneous phenotype is considered to be more severe in occurrence, has significantly a high rate of relapses and shorter first relapse-free survival time. Furthermore, the mucosal involvement at onset revealed a longer remission survival and may to impact the poor outcome of the disease. If it is difficult to achieve initial control (disease remission), patients are more likely to have a longer overall disease duration. In literature, it was documented that patients of ethnic group of Indo-Asian origin had substantially longer disease duration than Caucasian European patients. Furthermore, it was observed that remission survival was significantly longer in females than in males. Women may suffer from severe pemphigus vulgaris more frequently than men, more frequently they have multiple mucosal involvements. The genetic impact to the prognosis and outcome of pemphigus vulgaris was recently investigated. It was documented that carriers of one or both HLA DRB1* *04:02 and DQB1*05:03 produce significantly higher levels of anti -Dsg3 antibody than carriers of other HLA alleles. A recent study documented that patients carrying HLA DRB1*04:02 far more frequently revealed severe pemphigus vulgaris and more frequently have the mucocutaneous phenotype than those carrying other HLA alleles.

Chapter 2

DIAGNOSTICS IN PEMPHIGUS VULGARIS

ABSTRACT

The diagnosis of autoimmune bullous disease, including pemphigus vulgaris, is derived from clinical and histopathological features, direct immunofluorescence (DIF), indirect immunofluorescence (IIF), or enzyme-linked immunosorbent assay (ELISA). The titre of anti-Dsg antibodies may correlate with disease activity. DIF microscopy is considered a sensitive method for autoantibody detection in tissue, in active disease as well as in remission. Furthermore, DIF may link the immunological activity of the disease and may help in the management of pemphigus vulgaris. Until that time, therapy could be discontinued in patients with negative results of DIF after a long period of clinical remission. Only patients with negative results of circulating autoantibodies may benefit from a DIF study. On the other hand, patients with a higher anti-Dsg antibody titer are likely to experience pemphigus recurrence.

INTRODUCTION

The classification of autoimmune bullous dermatoses is still based on histopathological criteria, primarily according to the localization of blisters, namely intraepidermal in pemphigus diseases and subepidermal in the pemphigoid group and dermatitis herpetiformis. Immunopathological criteria of pemphigus diseases are divided into pemphigus vulgaris, pemphigus foliaceus, paraneoplastic pemphigus and IgA pemphigus. Pemphigus diseases are characterized by intraepidermal blister formation due to the loss of adhesion of keratinocytes, and they are associated with antibodies to the intercellular junctions of keratinocytes. Target antigens of autoantibodies have been identified. In general, the pathogenicity of autoantibodies has been conclusively demonstrated experimentally. There is a parallel stratification in different layers of the epidermis of the antigens targeted by autoantibodies in the two forms of pemphigus disease. Dsg1 is located predominantly in the superficial layers of the epidermis and is absent in the suprabasilar layer, whereas Dsg3 is located predominantly in the deeper layers and is absent in the most superficial layers. [425] Acantholytic keratinocytes are considered to be the key element for the histologic diagnosis. However, they are neither pathognomic for a particular disease, nor an exclusive feature of intraepidermal bullous disease.

For routine histological examination, a fresh vesicle or blister (less than 24 hrs old) is biopsied, preferably in its entirety, placed in formaldehyde, and processed for hematoxylin and eosin staining. For the DIF microscopy, the biopsy specimen is taken from perilesional (> 1 cm from the lesion) or uninvolved skin. [426] The biopsy must be immediately frozen in native form and stored at temperatures below -70°C or placed in a special transport medium termed Michel´s solution, which is suitable for later immunofluorescence testing. [427] Circulating serum autoantibodies can be performed by IIF microscopy on frozen sections of normal tissues, including human skin, monkey esophagus, and rodent or monkey bladder. Autoantibodies directed against different autoantigens that co-localize microscopically cannot be differentiated based on patterns obtained by IIF microscopy. However, identification of target antigen can be performed using immunoassays, including ELISA and Western blot. Both native antigens from skin extracts or cultured keratinocytes and different recombinant antigens are employed as substance for these immunoassays. Several forms of pemphigus have been described depending on the level of intraepidermal split, including two major subtypes, pemphigus vulgaris and pemphigus foliaceus. The splitting formation is suprabasilar in pemphigus vulgaris and in it´s rare vegetating form, pemphigus vegetans. Superficial blistering formation is localized in pemphigus foliaceus and related sub-types. [428]

HISTOPATHOLOGY

In pemphigus, the basic abnormality is the loss of keratinocyte adhesion, described as acantholysis. The localization of the cleft formed by acantholysis is different in pemphigus vulgaris and pemphigus foliaceus types. The fully developed pemphigus vulgaris lesion is characterized by the occurrence of intraepidermal spitting with a sparse inflammatory infiltrate. Split formation occurs immediately above the basilar layer of the epidermis, suprabasilarly, leaving a single layer of basilar keratinocytes attached to the dermal-epidermal membrane called "row of tombstones" (Figure 2.1). [314] However, in some patients the splitting is also localized in lower levels of the spinous layer. The blisters contain serum and acantholytic keratinocytes. Acantholytic cells are round and have intensive eosinophilic cytoplasm, a pyknotic nucleus, and a perinuclear halo (Figure 2.2) In older blisters, neutrophilic and eosinophilic granulocytes, lymphocytes and macrophages are seen with scant perivascular infiltrate. Older lesions, clinically erosions and ulcerations, may have several layers of keratinocytes at the base of the blister due to keratinocyte migration and proliferation. [429] In early lesions, eosinophilic or neutrophilic spongiosis is pronounced, even as the sole histological manifestation. [430] Eosinophilic and neutrophilic spongiosis is not specific for pemphigus vulgaris and it is also seen in various conditions, among them acute contact dermatitis, pemphigus foliaceus, bullous pemphigoid, drug eruption, and spongiotic reaction to insect bites. [431] Mucosal involvement in pemphigus vulgaris reveals histologically identical characteristics to that of skin lesions. In the oral cavity, it is difficult to observe blisters because they may frequently be hampered due to trauma or mastification. Thus, the biopsy specimen will only reveal erosions or ulcerations. Therefore, biopsy specimen from the oral cavity should preferably be obtained from the margin of a denuded area. This location may show specific histologic alterations.

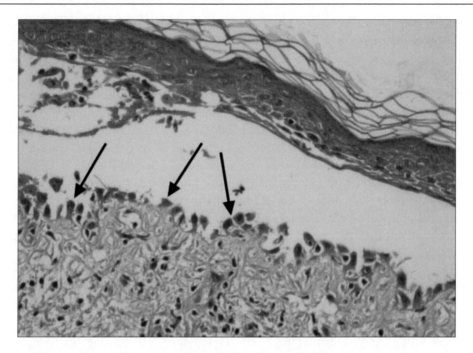

Figure 2.1. Histopathology of pemphigus vulgaris "row of tombstones."
"Tombstone" basilar cells (arrows) are localized at the base of the intraepidermal cleft. Inside the cleft are fibrin and acantholytic cells and neutrophilic leukocytes. Hematoxilin and eosin staining, 250x.

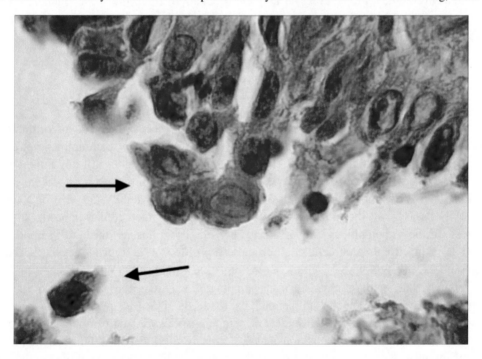

Figure 2.2. Histopathology of pemphigus vulgaris acantholytic cells.
Acantholytic cells (arrows) are localized inside of the intraepidermal cleft. Hematoxilin and eosin staining, 400x.

The histopathology of pemphigus vegetans, a subtype of pemphigus vulgaris, is similar to that of pemphigus vulgaris. However, it is a vegetative condition, revealing features of papillomatosis and acanthosis. In addition, microabscesses containing eosinophils can occasionally be observed. Moreover, a small number of dysplastic keratinocytes can be revealed. The histologic findings in the vegetating lesions are similar for both subtypes of pemphigus vegetans, of Hallopeau and Neumann subtypes. [428]

Cytology is a diagnostic method, based on investigation of the characteristics of individual cells. A cytology or Tzank test proves to be a very useful diagnostic tool in pemphigus diseases. This method was introduced by Arnault Tzanck in 1947. [432] Nowadays, it is replaced with other modern methods despite the many advantages such as simplicity, low cost, reliability, rapid preparation and relatively painless procedure. Moreover, multiple samples can be taken from different lesions and regions where taking a biopsy could be difficult. A fresh blister should be selected for sampling. The most common used stain is May-Grünwald -Giemsa. The others include Wright, Diff-Quack stain, Papanicolau, and hematoxylin and eosin. [432] Pemphigus diseases are characterized by numerous single or loosely adherent clumps of acantholytic cells. These cells are round in shape with a basophilic cytoplasm, especially at their periphery ("mourning-edged" cells). The nucleolus is hypertrophic and often shows atypical changes, but nucleoli are hazy and absent. By using immunocytofluorescence microscopy and treating the smear with fluoresceine anti-IgG antibody serum, pemphigus Tzank cells show a typical greenish fluoresce on the basilar membrane if they are isolated, or have a network-like fluorescence (the same as histological preparations) if they are grouped together. [433] The phenomena of cell adherence, so-called Sertoli´s rosette, is non-pathognomic to pemphigus, but frequently detected. [433]

DIRECT IMMUNOFLUORESCENCE MICROSCOPY

A histologic study alone is not sufficient to establish a precise diagnosis of pemphigus diseases. DIF is still considered the gold standard in the diagnostics of autoimmune bullous diseases, including pemphigus vulgaris. The location of the biopsy site is of key importance to achieve the best possible sensitivity. DIF is performed on a specimen taken from perilesional skin with normal appearing skin in the immediate vicinity (>1 cm) of a fresh blister. All diseases of the pemphigus group demonstrate intercellular deposits in the epidermis. In both pemphigus vulgaris and pemphigus foliaceus the DIF sample of perilesional skin reveals intercellular substance deposition in a typical net-like pattern (honeycomb like) of IgG with or without complement C3. [434, 435] While an accentuation of the suprabasilar epidermis is seen in pemphigus vulgaris, the accentuation of the subcorneal epidermis is detected in pemphigus foliaceus. [436] A punctuate or dot-like pattern is not frequently seen in DIF studies of pemphigus vulgaris and pemphigus foliaceus. This special type of reactant deposition may accompany a typical continuous intercellular pattern of immune reactants or can be rare only solitary. [437] Tissue -fixed autoantibodies are present in 80-95% of patients Figure 2.3. [168] In pemphigus vegetans DIF microscopy reveals deposits of IgG and complement C3 in the intercellular spaces of the epidermis. Both subtypes, of Hallopeau and Neumann are indistinguishable, and similar to pemphigus vulgaris. [428]

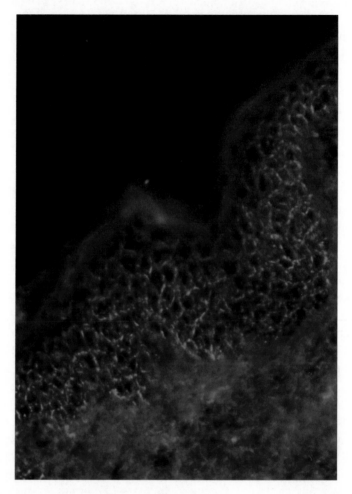

Figure 2.3. Direct immunofluorescence in pemphigus vulgaris.
Deposits of IgG are localized intercellularly in proportion to the whole epidermis (from the basilar layer up to the corneal layer). DIF IgG, 250x.

INDIRECT IMMUNOFLUORESCENCE MICROSCOPY

IIF microscopy is a screening method for circulating autoantibodies used in autoimmune blistering disease, including pemphigus group. All forms of pemphigus are associated with the presence of autoantibodies against keratinocyte cell-surface antigens. The IIF test is utilized to obtain titers of disease autoantibodies. Various substrates are used according to the subtypes of pemphigus. In pemphigus vulgaris and pemphigus foliaceus, guinea pig or monkey esophagus or human skin are the most sensitive substrates applied for detection of serum autoantibodies. To detect autoantibodies in plakin-rich tissue, e.g., in paraneoplastic pemphigus, rat or monkey bladder is the most appropriate substrate due to their high expression of plakins. [435] The pattern in IIF microscopy usually resembles those in DIF microscopy.

In pemphigus vegetans, the IIF method reveals IgG antibodies, identical to pemphigus vulgaris. [428]

Circulating pemphigus autoantibodies are present in about 80% of patients with active pemphigus disease and their titer usually correlates with disease activity. [166, 167, 438, 439]

TARGET ANTIGEN-SPECIFIC SEROLOGICAL ANALYSES OF PEMPHIGUS ANTIBODIES

ELISA (Enzyme-linked immunosorbent assay), Western blotting or immunopercipitation are highly sensitive and specific detection systems of autoantibodies utilizing recombinant autoantigens or keratinocyte extracts from human healthy skin. These tests are able to detect IgG or IgA against Dsg1, Dsg3, BP180, BP230, envoplakin, and are available commercially. [430] Immunoprecipitation is more difficult to perform and is generally less available then Western blotting. Unlike Western blotting, immunoprecipitation is performed with native, rather than denatured protein, and both are sensitive systems but time-consuming. Western blotting analyses are not useful in the diagnosis of pemphigus based on the fact that most of the epitopes on Dsg1 and Dsg3 are conformational. [430] On the other hand, ELISA possesses a quantitative method for measuring specific antibody levels utilizing recombinant human Dsg1 and Dsg3. Multiple ELISA assays are commercially available. The sensitivity of ELISA assay is very high. It was reported that sensitivity reached 100% for the diagnosis of pemphigus vulgaris and pemphigus foliaceus in untreated patients. When patients with systemic treatment were included, the sensitivity dropped to 95% in pemphigus vulgaris and 92% in pemphigus foliaceus. The high sensitivity of the ELISA assays was associated with a high specificity of 98%. [440, 441] Using a combination of Dsg1 and Dsg3 ELISA data, pemphigus vulgaris and pemphigus foliaceus could be distinguished. Recently, recombinant ectodomains of Dsg 1 and Dsg3 have been developed and used in highly sensitive and specific ELISA systems. The Dsg ectodomains are expressed in insect cells or in the human cell line HEK293. The sensitivity of the latter for anti-Dsg3 antibody was 100% and for anti-Dsg1 antibody was 95.6%. [167] The novel assay revealed a statistically significant relation between clinical severity and autoantibody levels in individual patients with pemphigus vulgaris and pemphigus foliaceus. Taken together, the ELISA systems are not only important tools for the diagnosis of pemphigus vulgaris and pemphigus foliaceus, but are also useful in monitoring serum autoantibody levels during the course of the disease. Circulating pemphigus autoantibodies are present in about 80% of patients with active pemphigus disease and their titer usually correlates with disease activity.

CONCLUSION

The diagnosis of pemphigus vulgaris is derived from clinical and histopathological features, direct immunofluorescence (DIF), indirect immunofluorescence (IIF), or enzyme-linked immunosorbent assay (ELISA). Titre of anti-Dsg antibodies may correlate with disease activity. ELISA systems are not only important tools for the diagnosis of pemphigus vulgaris, but are also useful in monitoring serum autoantibody levels during the course of the disease.

DIF microscopy is considered to be a very sensitive method for autoantibody detection in patients with pemphigus vulgaris in active disease and remission. Furthermore, it may link the immunological activity of the disease and may help in the management of pemphigus vulgaris. Until that time, therapy could be discontinued in patients with negative results of DIF after a long period of clinical remission. Authorities recommend that it is possible to discontinue immunosuppressive therapy in patients with pemphigus vulgaris who have revealed a DIF negative result if they are at least 6 months in clinical remission. [442] As the first step, an evaluation of serum autoantibody titer by IFF or ELISA should be performed. Only patients with negative results of circulating autoantibodies may benefit from a DIF study. On the other hand, patients with a higher anti-Dsg antibody titer are likely to experience pemphigus recurrence.

Chapter 3

CLINICAL CHARACTERISTICS OF PEMPHIGUS VULGARIS

ABSTRACT

The clinical characteristics of pemphigus vulgaris are well known, with the typical PV lesion being a blister. Most frequently, oral mucosa is the first appearance of pemphigus disease. The mucosa on sites other than the oral cavity is considered to be more commonly affected than was initially recorded. Nose, ocular, laryngeal, esophageal, genital and anal mucosa should be carefully examined using special assessment in cooperation with other specialists. Pemphigus vulgaris shows a variability of clinical picture developing through the outcome of the disease with remission and flares of clinical exacerbations. Recently, new scoring systems have been introduced, as follows: the autoimmune bullous skin disorder intensity score (ABSIS) and the pemphigus disease area index (PDAI), which may help in evaluating disease severity and its development.

INTRODUCTION

Pemphigus vulgaris represents a blistering disease that has an intraepidermal cleft in suprabasilar location of the epidermis depending on the pathophysiology of the disease.

Pemphigus vulgaris is the most frequent variant of pemphigus group, corresponding to 70-91% of all pemphigus cases. [5, 443] The disease manifests most frequently during middle age with an age peak between the 4th and 6th decade of life, less commonly it starts in the elderly or childhood. [444, 445]. Two major morphologic subtypes based on clinical and serologic criteria have been described in pemphigus vulgaris, the mucosal dominant and the mucocutaneous subtypes. Development of mucosal before cutaneous lesions is the most common in the mucocutaneous subtype. The mucosal membranes are usually involved first in about 80% of patients, especially in the oral mucosa. [446] A history of cutaneous -only phenotype in pemphigus vulgaris, which never had mucosal lesions, has only rarely been described, but is not unknown. In Eastern Sicily 36.5% (23/63) of patients with pemphigus vulgaris developed initial cutaneous lesions, and 22.2% (14/63) had exclusively skin manifestations and never had mucosal lesions. [13]

CLINICAL CHARACTERISTICS

Mucosal lesions in the oral cavity are flaccid blisters and soon after forming they leave erosions or ulcerated area. Although any surface can be involved, the most common sites are the buccal and labial mucosa, and the palate. Less frequently, the gingiva, floor of the mouth, posterior pharynx, and the tongue can be afflicted (Figure 3.1 and Figure 3.2). [447, 448] Fragile blisters are usually not seen because of permanent movement and mastication in the oral cavity. Erosions and the ulcerated area are typically painful. Denuded lesions are usually multiple, superficial and irregular in shape and arise from mucosa of healthy appearance. [148] Most patients complain of dysphagia and sometimes weight loss. The ulcerative lesions in the oral cavity do not heal, by contrast to other diagnoses located in this area, like aphtous stomatitis or stomatitis of viral origin. Oral involvement remains isolated for some months in most of the patients and frequently not recognized for a long time.

Skin involvement usually occurs after mucosal involvement. The flaccid and fragile blisters are replaced by weeping erosions followed by shiny or crusty appearance. Cutaneous lesions can occur on the entire skin surface, especially at the intertriginous site or at the site of mechanical irritation. During the active phase of pemphigus, both Nikolsky´s sign I and II can be elicited and aid clinical diagnosis. Nikolsky's sign I constitutes the perilesional separation of epidermis from dermis as a result of tangential pressure to the perilesional skin. [449] An additional less specific sign is Nikolsky's sign II, where an intact blister can be shifted laterally and enlarged by digital pressure. [450]

The disease is recognized most frequently after several months or longer, when the response to treatment fails. Pemphigus vulgaris should be considered in anyone who has multiple, non-healing oral erosions or ulcers that persist for longer than one month. [148] When the patients is not adequately treated, after several weeks or months, the condition progresses with lesions appearing on the scalp, face, and upper trunk and with affliction of other mucosa like nasal, pharyngeal, laryngeal, esophageal and genital and anal. Occasionally, the skin lesions occur as an initial manifestation of the disease. The initial small blisters are filled with a clear fluid and arise from normal appearing skin (Figure 3.3). After several days the blisters rupture leaving sharply outlined superficial erosions with a collarette of loose epidermis (Figure 3.4). Skin lesions are most frequently located on the upper trunk and scalp, involving the medial and central part rather than the sides. Although the scalp is frequently involved in pemphigus vulgaris, associated hair loss has only rarely been described. [451, 452] Other areas commonly afflicted are the face and neck. In some patients the periugual areas are involved, arising in loosening of the nail plate. [453] Generally, involvement of the nail is associated with severe and widespread disease. The condition is painful and cosmetically concerning. The healing is delayed and followed with recovery and growth of normal nail plate.

With treatment, skin lesions heal with crusting followed by re-epithelization and residual hyperpigmentation at sites of former lesions. This sign usually disappears in several months. Any scaring as sequelae is present in all pemphigus lesions.

Involvement of mucosa other than in the oral cavity can be seen in the esophagus, pharyngo-laryngeal mucosa, and genital or anal mucosa. The ENT endoscopy should be performed in all patients with pemphigus vulgaris, because it allows documenting of the real extent of disease involvement. Experts suggest that information related to traumatic physiological mechanisms on ear, nose and throat areas (mainly chewing, nose blowing, swallowing, phonation) must be offered to patients to avoid the appearance of new active lesions and to differentiate them from other entities, including candidal infection. Mucosal dysfunctions, swallowing, phonation, respiration, hearing and olfaction could be seen. Hoarseness or hemorrhagic crusts on the nasal mucosa, blood-tinged mucous and nasal obstruction can be observed. [454] Mucosal involvement other than in the oral cavity is present in the later course of the disease, in contrast to oral involvement which in majority of cases is the first manifestation of the disease. Laryngeal and nasal affliction is more frequent than usually believed. Several studies documented a high prevalence of pemphigus lesions in this location as followed with 13/16 (81%) involvement presented with throat symptoms, accounting for 12/16 (75%) patients with pharyngeal and 7/16 (44%) patients with laryngeal symptoms. [455] Another study referred about laryngeal and nasal involvement presented in 34/40 (85%) and 28/40 (70%) of patients with pemphigus vulgaris. [456] Contrary reports documented an association of mucosa involvement of the ear, nose and throat and severity and clinical involvement. One study reported that this mucosal involvement was not associated with severity and clinical involvement. [457] On the other hand, severe involvement of mucosa of the ear, nose and throat was associated with severity and clinical involvement in another study [33]. Despite this finding, patients with exclusively oropharyngeal localization have a more favorable course of the disease than those with mucocutaneous involvement. [458] A good outcome was also documented in a very rare case of exclusively laryngeal involvement. [459] The symptoms of laryngeal involvement in patients with pemphigus vulgaris are identical to those of candidiasis and therefore an ear, nose and throat assessment should be performed to differentiate these two conditions, which are treated very differently. The extension of pemphigus vulgaris lesions to the esophagus is relatively uncommon. One case series study documented eight cases with esophageal involvement in pemphigus vulgaris. [460] Esophageal lesions may be revealed by upper gastrointestinal endoscopy.

Another very rare localization is an ocular involvement (Figure 3.5). One study documented ocular involvement in 16.5% (17/103) of patients with pemphigus vulgaris. Conjunctiva was the most prevalent type of ocular involvement (9/17, 52.9%) followed by palpebral conjunctiva (7/17, 41.2%). [461] The ocular pemphigus is accompanied by photophobia and tearing. [462, 463] Ocular involvement results in complete recovery when treated and scarring is usually not sequelae.

In addition, the genital tract can be involved especially in females. Vulvar lesions occur more commonly than vaginal lesions and can be present at the initial disease presentation together with other mucosal sites involvement. The erosions are associated with a burning sensation and pain on micturition, and a foul odor. [464] Furthermore, cervical involvement is observed very rarely and can result in acantholytic cells being reported as an abnormal Pap smear, revealed in 26% (20/77) of female patients with pemphigus vulgaris. [465] The same study documented 51% (39/77) genital involvement in females. [465] This finding elucidates that genital involvement in females is more common than was previously thought. It is probably the second most common mucosal site of pemphigus vulgaris after oral mucosa. Involvement of penile skin is rare and when present it is associated with widespread disease. Lesions involving the penile skin were most commonly seen on the glans. [466] Genital involvement in both genders is healing with no sequelae or functional abnormalities. Less documented are anal lesions that can correlate with other mucosal involvement, especially with oral severe course of the disease. Constipation is the most frequent symptom followed by pain on defecation. In one study, 27.9% (47/168) of patients with pemphigus vulgaris were referred with anal involvement. [467] Anal involvement in patients with pemphigus vulgaris is probably more frequent than previously assumed. The details of involvement and comprehensive studies on ocular, vaginal, cervical or anal mucosa are still lacking.

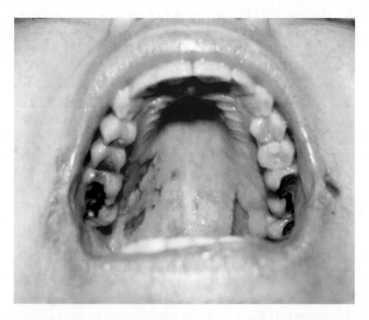

Figure 3.1. Oral pemphigus vulgaris. Erosions localized on the hard palate.

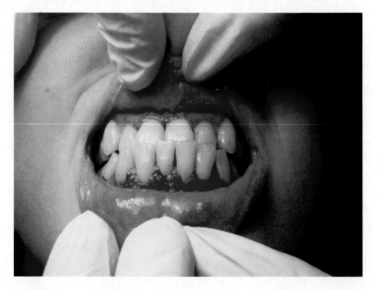

Figure 3.2. Oral pemphigus vulgaris.Erosions localized on the upper and lower gingiva.

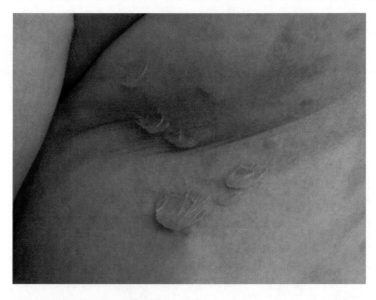

Figure 3.3. Pemphigus vulgaris on the skin. Blisters on the skin.

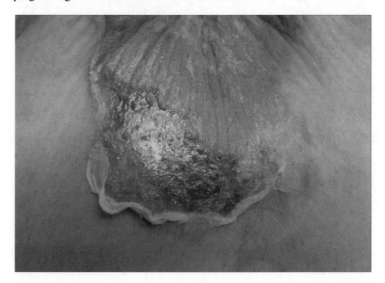

Figure 3.4. Pemphigus vulgaris on the skin. Ruptured blister with moist erosion. On the periphery of erosion is screwy epidermis.

In addition to pemphigus vulgaris, there is a rare variant pemphigus vegetans comprising only up to 1-2% of all pemphigus cases. [468] The type of pemphigus is considered to be less severe with better response to treatment. The predilection localization of pemphigus vegetans represents intertriginous spaces such as the groin, axillae and oral mucosa, as well as anogenital and nasolabial sites. Clinically, two subtypes are recognized: the Neumann type and Hallopeau type. They differ in their initial lesions. The Neumann type is characterized by flaccid blisters and erosions, whereas the Hallopeau type typically manifests with pustules. Blisters and pustules appear then in the course of time transform into extensive erosive areas. Both subtypes subsequently develop into hyperpigmented vegetative plaques, which are formed on erosions once the blisters rupture. At the periphery, hypertrophic granulation tissue or pustules are present. An intense fetid odor is present. [469] In more than half of the cases, the pemphigus vegetans begins in the oral cavity, often months before the appearance of skin lesions. In Neumann type, the oral lesions resemble those of pemphigus vulgaris. However, the blister-forming tendency is lower than in pemphigus vulgaris. The Neumann type, with worse prognosis than the Hallopeau type, is characterized by vegetation developing during the course of pemphigus vulgaris. [470] The Hallopeau type has a more benign course and few relapses. In addition, a characteristic feature of pemphigus vegetans is a cerebriform tongue, characterized by a pattern of sulci and gyri on the dorsum of the tongue. [449]

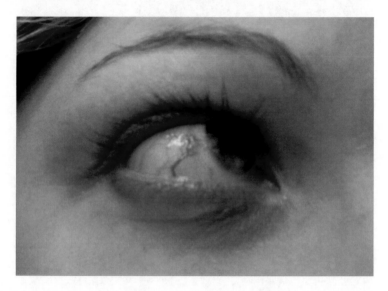

Figure 3.5. Ocular pemphigus vulgaris. Chronic conjunctivitis with hypertrophic and inflamed conjunctiva.

Pemphigus vulgaris shows a variability of clinical picture developing through the outcome of the disease with remission and flares of clinical exacerbations. In addition, the response to treatment management may differ from case to case. Various scoring systems were used to evaluate the severity of the disease and the response to treatment. Recently, new scoring systems are introduced as follows: the autoimmune bullous skin disorder intensity score (ABSIS) and the pemphigus disease area index (PDAI), which may help in evaluating disease severity and its development.

The first used evaluating score is the BSA (body surface area) which is often used in outcome measures to estimate the extent of disease development. [471] This score may underestimate disease severity that is localized on a small area of the body. The ABSIS skin score aims to measure the phenotypical varieties seen across pemphigus vulgaris, with careful consideration of skin and mucosal involvement as separate entities with different significance. The ABSIS skin score measures the extent of afflicted area and the quality of skin lesions. Extent is assessed by the percent of involvement BSA and the "rule of nine". Quality is assessed in three values as re-epithelialized lesions, erosive dry lesions, or erosive, exudative lesions with or without a positive Nikolsky's sign. The ABSIS skin score is calculated by multiplying the BSA by the appropriate quality-weighting factor. Oral involvement is assessed separately with two scores. The first score assesses the extent of the disease, assigning the presence of lesions into 11 distinct anatomical locations in the oral cavity. The second score measures the severity of oral lesions based on quality of pain/bleeding associated with certain foods. [472] The advantage of the ABSIS score is that it may evaluate both quantitative and qualitative information about skin and oral involvement. Another outcome measure is PDAI score which was developed by the International Pemphigus Committee. This evaluating system comprises three components relating to the skin, scalp and mucous membranes. The skin lesions are evaluated by activity and damage scores. The activity score is measured by the number of lesions at the time of examination. An individual activity score provides a value from 12 anatomic locations. The damage score valuates post-inflammatory hyperpigmentation or erythema from resolving lesions. A similar approach for 12 parts of the mucous membranes results in a mucous membrane severity score. [471] The PDAI score is able to detect smaller differences in severity in moderate-to-severe pemphigus than the ABSIS score. [473] Another advantage of the PDAI score is that this system accounts also mucous membranes of the body, including the anogenital area, eyes and nose mucosa. In addition, the post-inflammatory damage helps evaluate the severity of disease. These two scoring systems may be considered reliable tools to use in clinical trials due to their accuracy in assessing small differences in patients with pemphigus disease, as well as to evaluate treatment efficacy and can be used as a means of comparing various therapeutic options. Future multicenter studies investigating a larger number of patients with variable disease activities are essential in order to finally valuate the differences of those two scoring systems.

CONCLUSION

The clinical characteristics of pemphigus vulgaris are well known, but the mucosa on other sites than the oral cavity should be carefully examined using special assessment in cooperation with other specialists. It seems that other localities than oral mucosa are more frequently affected than recorded, including nose, ocular, laryngeal, esophageal, genital and anal mucosa. PDAI and ABSIS scoring systems may help in evaluating disease severity, efficacy of treatment and disease development.

Chapter 4

MANAGEMENT OF PEMPHIGUS VULGARIS

ABSTRACT

Management of pemphigus vulgaris should be started with an evaluation of disease severity. The patient´s overall medical condition should be evaluated for whether there is a large risk of developing complications from immunosuppressive treatment. Corticosteroids are the mainstay therapy in pemphigus vulgaris, which is lifesaving but accompanied by multiple side and adverse effects. Adjuvant therapy is used to reduce the total dose of corticosteroids and to increase their immunosuppression. Rapidly acting adjuvant therapies are used to control active disease. They include IVIG, plasmapheresis and immunoadsorption and rituximab; all of them are considered to be the second line of pemphigus therapy. Slowly acting adjuvant therapies are used during maintenance and/or consolidation phases of treatment in order to reduce the dose of corticosteroids. The choice of a particular agent is based on the physician's experience and the patient´s underlying medical condition, and the relative possibility of an undesirable side-effect profile. The group of adjuvant therapies with slow onset of action includes azathioprine, cyclophosphamide, cyclosporine, methotrexate, mycophenolate mofetil and anti-inflammatory drugs (e.g., dapsone, antimalarials, gold and tetracyclines). These medications are used in conjunction with systemic corticosteroids. The goal of the therapy is to induce complete remission with minimum side effects, allowing all therapy to be discontinued or the use of the lowest drug doses that prevent disease activation. Topical management disclosed new medications that promote healing, including topical immunomodulatory agents. Lesions in the oral cavity are frequently slow responding to systemic therapy. Medications that promote healing in the oral cavity used until now in oncology may augment management in pemphigus oral lesions.

INTRODUCTION

Pemphigus vulgaris is a rare chronic autoimmune disease with unpredictable course, despite new effective modalities of therapy used in its management. The advent of systemic immunosuppressants has considerably improved the prognosis of patients with pemphigus vulgaris. The goal of therapy is to achieve complete remission of skin and mucosal lesions. Systemic corticosteroids are the most useful drugs in treating pemphigus vulgaris, rapidly inducing remission in the majority of patients. Before the advent of corticosteroids, the diagnosis of pemphigus vulgaris carried such a poor prognosis that if a patient survived for more than 1 year, the diagnosis of pemphigus was often questioned. The introduction of corticosteroids in the 1950s dramatically reduced mortality from around 70% to 30%. The establishment of adjuvant immunosuppressive agents in the 1960s cut mortality to 10%. [474] Nowadays, it is estimated that mortality ranges from 5% to 10%. [5] Nevertheless, increased morbidity is associated with long-term administration of immunosuppressants, especially those of corticosteroids, including diabetes, hypertension, osteoporosis, sepsis and others.

MANAGEMENT OF PEMPHIGUS VULGARIS

Before treatment is initiated, the diagnosis should be confirmed by clinical, histological, and immunofluorescence data. Oral mucosa is the first to be evaluated and all other mucosal sites including the pharynx, larynx and the nasal cavity should be assessed by ENT examination if there are symptoms to suggest involvement in these areas. Other mucosal areas with involvement or symptoms should be assessed by special assessment, like a pelvic examination in the genital area of women, endoscopic examination of the esophagus and rectoscopic examination in anal symptoms. Before the initiation of therapy, it is recommended to investigate the complete blood cell count and differential, hematocrit, serum electrolytes and the level of urea, creatinine, liver function tests, and fasting glucose test. If azathioprine is to be used, assessment of the thiopurine methyl transferase concentration should be investigated. If dapsone is to be used, the reticulocyte count, glucose-6-phosphate dehydrogenase and methemoglobin level are to be examined. [426] The patient´s overall medical status should be evaluated for whether there is a great risk of developing complications from immunosuppressive treatment.

Corticosteroids are lifesaving and complications such as diabetes, hypertension, duodenal ulcers, cataracts, osteoporosis, psychiatric illness and other risk factors, mandate closer observation and the use of preventive measures. Adjuvant therapy may reduce the total dose of corticosteroids. There are several adjuvant therapies with a different mode of efficacy and speed of action. Rapidly acting adjuvant therapies are used to control active disease that is unresponsive to systemic corticosteroids. They include megadose pulse corticosteroids given intravenously, IVIG, plasmapheresis and immunoadsorption. The effectiveness of rapidly acting therapies is achieved within days to a few weeks. Slowly acting adjuvant therapies are used during maintenance and/or consolidation phases of treatment in order to reduce the dose of corticosteroids. Their effectiveness starts after 4-6 weeks of administration. The choice of a particular agent is based on the physician's experience and the patient´s underlying medical condition, and the relative possibility of an undesirable side-effect profile. The group of adjuvant therapy with slow onset of action includes cyclophosphamide, azathioprine, cyclosporine, methotrexate, mycophenolate mofetil and anti-inflammatory drugs (e.g., dapsone, antimalarials, gold and tetracyclines). These medications are used in conjunction with systemic corticosteroids.

Latent infection, including tuberculosis, should be examined with a tuberculin test and chest radiograph before the start of immunosuppressive therapy. If present, prophylactic therapy should be administered. Baseline bone density and ophthalmologic examination should be undertaken and repeated periodically while the patients are on corticosteroids.

The goal of the therapy is to induce a complete remission with minimum side effects that permits all therapy to be discontinued or the use of the lowest drug doses that prevent disease activation. Treatment of pemphigus vulgaris is divided into three phases, based on activity of the disease. The first is the control phase, followed by the consolidation phase and then the maintenance phase. [475] The control phase of treatment is the period in which the disease activity is suppressed usually by a high dose of immunosuppressant agent. There is no evidence of a pronounced reduction or complete suppression of new lesion formation and the beginning of lesion healing. The length of the control phase is measured in weeks, not months. Pemphigus vulgaris usually responds to treatment within two weeks, provided the correct dose is used. A continued control phase indicates an inadequate dose of medication or a complicated factor. In the consolidation phase, the dose of medication controls the disease and is maintained until the bulk of lesions have healed. The duration of this phase is also weeks, not months. Slow healing means the intensity of therapy is inadequate and should be increased. The doses of medication should not be tapered until most lesions (about 80%) have healed, so as to reduce the chance of a subsequent flare in disease activity. The maintenance phase begins once most lesions have healed. In the maintenance phase, the medication is gradually tapered to the lowest level that suppresses the appearance of new lesions, with the goal being to discontinue all medications eventually. If a patient is treated with multiple drugs, these should be tapered one at a time. Tapering too rapidly increases the chance of relapse, while tapering too slowly may lead to side effects of the medication. One can recommend reducing the prednisone dose by about a quarter every one to two weeks and the gradual conversion to an alternate day schedule once the daily dose is at 10-8 mg. The rate of medication tapering is based on the clinical manifestation of the disease and the physician's experience. If the serum level of autoantibodies does not continue to fall or new lesions (one to five) appear while medication is being tapered, these lesions can be treated with intralesional or high potency topical corticosteroid, while maintaining the patients on their current dose of systemic medications. [148] If many new lesions appear, the dose of corticosteroids should be increased in 25-50% increments until control of the disease is achieved. If the clinical manifestation achieved clearance of the skin and mucosal areas and the level of autoantibodies disappears, and also DIF data prove negative, the medication can be discontinued. However, discontinuation of the medication can ultimately be compassed in the majority of patients. The proportion of patients in whom discontinuation of immunosuppressive therapy can be achieved increases steadily with time, and it can be discontinued approximately in 50% of patients after 3 years and in 75% of patients after 10 years. [476, 477]

A lack of well-designed studies to evaluate the stage of disease and effectiveness of therapy resulted in the establishment of a consensus statement on definition, end point and therapeutic response for pemphigus vulgaris that has been defined in International Pemphigus Committee Meetings and published in 2008. [478] Some observation points could be used also in the practical management of PV patients. For example, control of disease activity (early endpoint) is defined as the time interval at which new lesions cease to form and established lesions begin to heal. This is also considered the beginning of the consolidation phase.

However, end of the consolidation phase means that no new lesions have developed for at least two weeks and the majority (approximately 80%) of established lesions has healed. At this point, most physicians begin to taper doses of medication. A late endpoint of disease activity is identified as complete remission off therapy and complete remission on therapy, whereby in both cases the patients have had no new or established lesions for at least 2 months. In complete remission on therapy, the patient receives minimal therapy, i.e., less than or equal to 10 mg/day of prednisone (or equivalent) and/or minimal adjuvant therapy for at least two months. Minimal adjuvant therapy is defined as half the dose required to be defined as treatment failure (see below). Partial remission of therapy is defined as the presence of transient new lesions that heal within one week without treatment and while the patient has been off all systemic therapies for at least two months. Partial remission on minimal therapy is defined as the presence of transient new lesions that heal within one week while the patient receives minimal therapy, including topical medication. A relapse of disease or a flare represents the appearance of three or more new lesions a month that do not heal spontaneously within one week, or an extension of established lesions in a patient who has achieved disease control. In some patients receiving a full dose of corticosteroids or adjuvant agent, failure of therapy can be seen with an undesirable response to the medication. The patients continue to develop new lesions or old lesions continue to extend, or established lesions fail to begin to heal despite three weeks off therapy on 1.5 mg/kg/day of prednisone equivalent with/without any of the following adjuvant agents administered for at least 12 weeks: cyclophosphamide 2 mg/kg/day, azathioprine 2.5 mg/kg/day, methotrexate 20 mg/week, and mycophenolate mofetil 3mg/day. [478] Methotrexate and mycophenolate mofetil doses are based on a 75 kg individual. Table 4.1. modified from ref. [481]

Table 4.1. Therapeutic algorithm in pemphigus vulgaris

First line treatment	Initial dose	Comments
Prednisone (Prednisolone)	0.5-1.5 mg/kg/day	Optimal dose not validated
First line adjuvant		
Azathioprine	1-3 mg /kg/day	TMP activity evaluated prior to treatment
Mycophenolate mofetil	2g/day	
Mycofenolic acid	1440 mg/day	
Second line treatment		
Intravenous immunoglobulins	2g/kg/month	Exclude IgA deficiency prior to treatment
Immunoadsorption	2 cycles a 4 days	(2.5-fold total plasma volume/d), 4 weeks apart
Rituximab	2 x 1 g i.v.	2 weeks apart ; exclude hypersensitivity to mouse proteins
	4x 375 mg/m2	Each 1 week apart
Cyclophosphamide	500 mg i.v. bolus	Secondary sterility, hemorhagic cystitis
	2 mg /kg/day orally	and secondary cystic cancer
Dapsone	100 mg/day	Glucoso-6-phosphate dehydrogenase
	1.5 mg/kg/day	acitivity evaluated prior to treatment
Methotrexate	10-20 mg /week	Substitute folate 5-15 mg on the following day

Topical therapy is used to keep lesions clean and reduce pain, and also to prevent and treat secondary infections that can delay the response to therapy. [148] Most patients are treated with systemic corticosteroids, which display good efficacy. Adjuvant drugs are commonly used in combination with corticosteroids to increase their immunosuppressive efficacy and so to reduce their dose. The adjuvant agent corticosteroid-sparing effect lets the maintenance dose of corticosteroids be reduced and their side effects avoided. Despite this, some studies reported that patients treated with corticosteroids alone demonstrated outcomes comparable with those of using adjuvant drugs. [479] The effectiveness of adjuvant drugs was not exactly confirmed by prospective, controlled studies that conclusively demonstrate the benefits of adjuvant drugs in pemphigus vulgaris. Some respected authorities therefore use adjuvant drugs, unless there are contraindications or side effects of corticosteroids, or if tapering of the dose is accompanied by repeated relapses. [474]

The duration of different treatment regimens is not standardized, ranging from 1 to 5 years or even longer. Prolonged treatment duration leads to high cumulative doses of corticosteroids and adjuvant drugs. In general, minimizing potential side effects of corticosteroid therapy is considered by using agents that reduce osteoporosis, antancids, and by encouraging exercise, following a diet low in sugar and salt, and by minimizing dental procedures, sun exposure and radiation therapy, which all can cause a flare in disease activity. [475] Such supported therapy and measures to prevent side effects in adjuvant drugs are recommended in all potential regimens of treating pemphigus vulgaris.

Physicians and patients alike should be aware that pemphigus vulgaris may not require lifelong treatment. To date, very few studies have used the end points proposed by the consensus statement. However, the rate of patients achieving complete remission off therapy reflects the rate of patients who heal from their disease. The prognostic factors of complete remission off therapy are still unknown. It is believed that factors such as initial disease severity, type of pemphigus vulgaris, or initial treatment regimen may all influence the rate of complete remission off therapy. Hitherto, there is still no confirmed "best treatment strategy" for pemphigus vulgaris. This may be due to the disease's rarity, to the fact that it has various phenotypes, and to its variable severity. Still, there are controversies on the opportunity of adjuvant immunosuppressive drugs. For some, they are just steroid-sparing drugs. For others, they are disease modifying drugs.

However, the management of pemphigus vulgaris must take into account the disease's impact on various aspects of the patient's life, including physical, emotional and functional involvement, which should be considered before deciding on the optimal therapeutic protocol. The side effects are more frequently registered in older individuals with a positive medical history for diabetes and /or cardiovascular disorders and other serious conditions. The patient's physical profile, including concomitant diseases and medication, as well as certain demographic characteristics (especially age) at baseline, should therefore be taken into consideration before deciding on the final therapeutic scheme.

CORTICOSTEROIDS

Corticosteroids have anti-inflammatory and immunosuppressive efficacy. Their effects arise from suppressing the production of proinflammatory mediators by many cells of the immune system, including macrophages, monocytes, endothelial cells, basophils, fibroblasts, and lymphocytes. The therapeutic effect is also mediated by direct anti-acantholytic action of corticosteroids that protects keratinocytes from an autoantibody-induced damage. [480]

Corticosteroids are the mainstay in management of pemphigus vulgaris due to their rapid effects, resulting in a significant improvement in the morbidity and mortality rates. The optimum dosing schedule is empirical and based on practical experience. Some dermatologic authorities recommend an initial dose equivalent to 0.5-1.5 mg of prednisolone/kg daily, which is often sufficient to control disease activity. [481] The dosing schedule is advocated according to disease severity and a modified regimen is suggested. Patients with mild disease are treated with initial prednisolone doses of 40-60 mg daily, and more severe cases with 60-100 mg daily. [482] If the patient does not respond within 5-7 days, the dose should be increased in 50-100% increments until there is disease control. When patients do not respond well to systemic prednisolone therapy even at higher doses, the change of prednisolone to other oral corticosteroid (e.g., bethamethasone, dexamethasone or methylprednisolone) may improve the patient's condition. [483] A clinical improvement may be seen within days of starting corticosteroids. On average, the cessation of blistering takes 2-3 weeks and full healing may be observed in 6-8 weeks. [484] Autoantibody titers fall with corticosteroids and clinical improvement, but the decrease in autoantibody titers is slower than the clinical improvement. Once remission is induced with healing of the majority of lesions (about 80%), the dose of medication should be tapered. A 50% reduction every 2 weeks has been suggested. [474] Another opinion is to reduce the dose by 5-10 mg of prednisolone a week and more slowly below 20 mg of prednisolone daily. [481]

In severe and recalcitrant disease, a daily dose above 100 mg is required. In these cases, intravenous pulsed therapy should be administered. [485] The theoretical aim of pulsing is to achieve more rapid and effective disease control compared with conventional oral dosing, thus allowing a reduction in long-term maintenance doses and their side effects. Doses of pulse therapy are not standardized but are usually 10 to 20 mg/kg for methylprednisolone (250-1000 mg) or 2 to 5 mg/kg (50-200 mg) for dexamethasone. These very high doses, sometimes termed megadoses, are usually administered as intravenous infusions over 30 minutes to 1 hour daily for a total of 1 to 5 administrations. [474] In most indications, pulse therapy is followed by the continuous administration of a low or intermediate dose of corticosteroid and/or adjuvant immunosuppressive agents. [486] Intravenous pulsed therapy is especially recommended in patients with a fresh onset of severe or recalcitrant disease. However, adverse effects are common and dose related. Complication from treatment can result from either acute withdrawal or prolonged use. Acute withdrawal may result in acute adrenal insufficiency. The condition could be serious and is characterized by fever, malaise, myalgias, arthralgias, and rarely, pseudotumor cerebri. [487]

The threat of side and adverse effects in systemic corticosteroids is high because mostly all patients with pemphigus vulgaris are dependent on systemic therapy. Long-term and high dose treatment with systemic corticosteroids carries a high risk of serious adverse effects, however, including fluid and electrolyte imbalance (hypokalemia, edema and hypertension), hyperglycemia and diabetes, peptic ulceration, weight gain, increased susceptibility to infections, proximal myopathy, behavioral changes (insomnia, nervousness, mood changes and psychosis), Cushing's syndrome and ophthalmologic complications such as cataracts. During a 20-year follow-up period, side effects of corticosteroids were documented in 81.8% (36/44) of patients with pemphigus vulgaris. The most common side effect was osteopenia and osteoporosis in 59.1% (26/44) of patients, followed by cataract (52%, 23/44). [33] In addition, other side effects may be associated, such as hirsutizm, abdominal straie, menstrual irregularity, purpura, hypopigmentation, cutaneous atrophy and impaired wound healing, severe infections and thromboembolic complications. Among these adverse effects, a severe bacterial infection may cause a very serious condition associated with disseminated intravascular coagulation or sepsis and can be life-threatening. The development of osteoporosis is strictly dose related and associated with the duration of therapy. It is estimated that in 30% to 50% of patients on a long-term regimen develop fractures of the trabecular bone or the vertebral bodies. [488] Patients receiving long-term therapy are recommended to undergo baseline bone densitometry; especially postmenopausal women, while this should be repeated at 1 to 2-year intervals. Supporting the administration of calcium (1.500 mg/day), vitamin D (400 IU/day), and biphosphonates such as alendronate is necessary in order to avoid complication such as osteonecrosis (avascular necrosis) of the femoral and humeral head, as well as of the distal portion of the femur. Ophthalmologic examinations should be assessed regularly to screen for cataracts and glaucoma. [488] Because of side and adverse effects, the goal in the management of patients with pemphigus vulgaris is to reduce the patient´s cumulative exposure to systemic corticosteroids.

In the long list of immunosuppressants recommended for treatment of pemphigus vulgaris, corticosteroids remain the mainstay despite their frequent and numerous side and adverse effects.

Adjuvant Drugs

Adjuvant drugs are usually administered in combination with systemic corticosteroids so as to reduce related side effects and increase the drug efficacy. Recently, adjuvant immunosuppressants and immunomodulators have been applied as initial treatment in combination with corticosteroids in order to decrease the initial dose of corticosteroids. Azathioprine, cyclosporine, mycophenolate mofetil and cyclophosphamide have been used. The adverse effects of each drug are different, but myelosuppression, abnormal data in liver function tests, jaundice, kidney dysfunction, malignancies, and infection, are common in all of them. When the disease improves, dosage should be tapered prior to that of the immunosuppressant. In literature, there is no clearly defined benefit of immunosuppressive drug combination. There are even some reports that show a higher incidence of complications with combination therapy (prednisolone and cyclophosphamide, or prednisolone and cyclosporine). [489] Another report referred the mean time to induce remission as shorter in the high dose oral prednisolone monotherapy than in low dose oral prednisolone on alternate days, plus azathioprine every day. [490] Rapidly progressive lesions necessitate a high prednisolone dose for early and adequate control of the disease. However, the significantly higher mean dose is directly correlated to an increased rate of treatment-associated adverse events. In terms of early disease control and rapid disease regression, monotherapy with corticosteroid seems to be superior to combination therapy corticosteroid plus azathioprine. [491] Another study referred that the efficacy of corticosteroid is enhanced when combined with a cytotoxic drug. Azathioprine is usually well tolerated and is generally believed to be more effective than prednisolone alone, both in terms of mortality and morbidity. [492] Azathioprine seems to be the most efficacious cytotoxic drug to reduce corticosteroids, followed by cyclophosphamide (used as pulse therapy) and mycophenolate mofetil. [492]

Azathioprine

Azathioprine is the best characterized first-line immunosuppressive and corticosteroid-sparing agent for treatment of pemphigus vulgaris. Azathioprine is a purine analog and is non-enzymatically converted to 6-mercaptopurine after oral administration and absorption. Azathioprine and 6-mercaptopurine are both pro-drugs. The 6-mercaptopurine is activated by several enzymatic steps to its active metabolites, 6-thioguanine nucleotides, and can be inactivated by xanthine oxidase to 6-thiouric acid, or by thiopurine methyltransferase (TPMT) to 6-methyl-mercaptopurine. The activity of TPMT is genetically determined and may be associated with gene polymorphism. Approximately 10% of the population has a heterozygote genotype with intermediate enzyme activity, and about 1 in 300 patients is homozygous for mutant alleles or is heterozygous with low enzyme activity. [493] Patients with insufficiency of TPMT may experience rapid bone marrow suppression after initiation of azathioprine treatment. Assessing TPMT activity before initiating azathioprine therapy is recommended so as to disclose its deficiency. Furthermore, some patients may experience this complication despite normal TPMT activity. All patients at risk of severe toxicity should undergo close monitoring of clinical and hematologic parameters. In addition, an abrupt increase in transaminase levels in serum observed soon after administration of azathioprine is a clue for deficient TPMT activity. Likewise, concurrent therapy with TPMT-inhibiting drugs, such as allopurinol or sulfasalazine, can also increase the risk of myelotoxicity. [493] In addition to its effects on nucleic acid synthesis, azathioprine also affects the immune system. Azathioprine is thought to be relatively specific to lymphocytes and is more selective for T cells than B cells. [494] Since azathioprine interferes with purine synthesis and metabolism, the disruption in such a fundamental level may explain its delay of action, as it usually takes at least 1 to 2 months before clinical effects are seen. [495]

Adverse drug reactions to azathioprine occur in 15% to 30% of patients and include leucopenia, thrombocytopenia, anemia, pancytopenia and hepatotoxicity. Long-lasting immunosuppression increases the risk of infections and only a small increase of neoplasia, mostly lymphoma. [494] In addition, alopecia, erythematous or maculopapular rash or gastrointestinal problems (nausea, vomiting, anorexia, diarrhea, aphthous stomatitis and pancreatitis) can be observed. In pregnancy, azathioprine is contraindicated due to its risk to the fetus; the same is referred for breastfeeding, because a minimal concentration of the drug and its metabolites has been discovered in breast milk. [495]

In autoimmune bullous disorders, including pemphigus vulgaris, the recommended dosage of azathioprine is 1 to 3 mg/kg daily, adjusted within these limits according to response. [481] The lowest effective dosage is administered. If no improvement occurs in the patient's condition within 3 months, consideration should be given to withdrawing azathioprine. However, with good efficacy, care should be taken in monitoring for myelosuppression and possible hepatotoxicity. The data sheet for azathioprine recommends weekly monitoring of a full blood count for the first 8 weeks of treatment, then at a minimum of once every 3 months. Routine monitoring also includes liver function tests. It is therefore advised to monitor weekly blood count and liver function tests until the maintenance dose is achieved, followed by regular monitoring, reducing to a minimum of once every 3 months for the duration of therapy. [494] More frequent monitoring of blood tests is advised in patients with hepatic or renal impairment, in the elderly, and in those treated with high doses of azathioprine.

The administration of live vaccines to patients receiving azathioprine is contraindicated and a diminished response to killed vaccines may occur. [496] An increased risk of serious infection, including sepsis, can be seen foremost in patients treated with a combination of corticosteroids and azathioprine. [497] The sudden onset of abdominal pain, with or without vomiting, may be due to pancreatitis related to the azathioprine treatment. The serum amylase should be checked urgently in these patients. A randomized double blind study of prednisolone and azathioprine in 56 patients with pemphigus vulgaris documented the corticosteroid-sparing effect of azathioprine. [491] Extensive experience with azathioprine refers to good efficacy, tolerability and safety, and the drug is recommended as an adjuvant corticosteroid-sparing immunosuppressant in the first line. Precise monitoring of blood tests may prevent suspected adverse effects.

Mycophenolate Mofetil

Mycophenolate mofetil, or its active metabolite mycophenolic acid, is a selective inhibitor of inosine monophosphate dehydrogenase in purine synthesis, required for T cell and B cell growth. The result of activity is the suppression of lymphocyte proliferation by inhibiting *de novo* purine synthesis. This suppression results in decreased antibody production. Because mycophenolate mofetil specifically inhibits the *de novo* pathway, lymphocytes are the primary target of mycophenolate mofetil action *in vivo*, thereby minimizing unwanted effects on other cell types. [498]

Mycophenolate mofetil is a relatively new agent in therapy of pemphigus vulgaris. Originally, it was developed for the treatment of psoriasis and tumors. Mycophenolate mofetil has been approved for acute renal transplant rejection due to its immunosuppressive effects exerted primarily on lymphocytes. [498] There is great individual variability in the kinetics and metabolism of mycophenolate. Mycophenolate mofetil in combination with prednisolone produces an effective drug in the treatment of pemphigus vulgaris. [499] The usual dose of mycophenolate mofetil is 0.5 to 2 g per day or mycophenolic acid (1440 mg/day). [481] The induction of disease remission often requires at least 8 weeks of treatment. Mycophenolate mofetil is generally well-tolerated and serious adverse effects were rarely observed. Adverse effects include diarrhea, nausea, vomiting, infections, leucopenia, or anemia, or both. It´s safety profile is characterized by a low toxicity causing only moderate adverse effects. Hematologic findings are dose-related and reversible and include anemia, leucopenia, and thrombocytopenia. Intravenous administration is commonly associated with thrombophlebitis and thrombosis. [496] There is a small increase of infections, especially herpes zoster. Infrequent adverse effects can include esophagitis, gastritis, gastrointestinal tract hemorrhage, or invasive cytomegalovirus infection. The drug is contraindicated in pregnancy because of the increased risk of miscarriage and congenital malformations. [498]

Mycophenolate mofetil is considered in recalcitrant cases of pemphigus vulgaris or when azathioprine and cyclophosphamide cannot be used. [499] In one comparative study of corticosteroid plus adjuvant such as azathioprine or mycophenolate mofetil in the treatment of pemphigus vulgaris, both demonstrated similar efficacy, sparing effect and safety profiles. [500] Because of its´ good effectiveness and appropriate safety profile, mycophenolate mofetil could replace azathioprine as an antimetabolite adjuvant of choice in the treatment of many autoimmune and inflammatory diseases, including pemphigus vulgaris. Recently, mizoribine, another purine biosynthesis inhibitor, was developed and has low toxicity. The pharmacological effects of mizoribine are similar to those of mycophenolate mofetil. [501] It was discovered in Japan and utilized for the treatment of diseases such as renal transplantation, rheumatoid arthritis and lupus nephritis. [502] There are only small group-based reports of mizoribine efficacy in autoimmune bullous diseases, including pemphigus vulgaris. In a small number of patients with pemphigus vulgaris, mizoribine demonstrated good efficacy and safety and enabled a substantial reduction in the corticosteroid dose. [503]

Cyclophosphamide

Cyclophosphamide is an immunosuppressive agent that alkylates DNA at various sites, resulting in cell cycle arrest, DNA repair, and apoptosis. [487] Proliferating tissues with a high mitotic rate are the most susceptible. However, its' activity is not cell cycle-dependent. The toxicity is significantly higher than that of azathioprine. Adverse effects are frequent, including acute myelosuppression, which can be developed at 6 to 10 days and recovered in 14 to 21 days. [487] Both cellular and humoral immunity are suppressed. In addition, other adverse effects can be present, including mucosal ulcers, nausea and vomiting, stomach pain, diarrhea, nephrotoxicity, urotoxicity (hemorrhagic cystitis), cardiotoxicity, hepatotoxicity (venous occlusive disease), interstitial lung fibrosis, darkening of the skin and nails, alopecia, changes in color and texture of the hair, and lethargy. Cyclophosphamide can seriously attack reproductive systems in both genders, resulting in amenorrhea that is often permanent and azoospermia that is often irreversible. [487] Cyclophosphamide is mutagenic and carcinogenic. Its long-term administration can be associated with acute non-lymphocytic leukemia.

Several studies referred the corticosteroid-sparing effect of cyclophosphamide at oral doses of 50-200 mg daily in case series or 2mg/kg/day. [481, 504, 505] Thus, when azathioprine fails to produce remission or a corticosteroid-sparing effect, cyclophosphamide may be an effective alternative. Results of one study on a small number of patients indicated that an initial combined program of cyclophosphamide and prednisolone may be a highly effective treatment for pemphigus vulgaris. In some cases, prolonged remission with cessation of all therapy was possible. [506] Pulsed intravenous cyclophosphamide can be administered in combination with dexamethasone or methylprednisolone. The regimen consists of the intermittent administration of a high dose of intravenous corticosteroid and cyclophosphamide, usually as three daily doses of corticosteroid (dexamethasone 100 mg or methylprednisolone 500-1000 mg) and a single dose of cyclophosphamide (500 mg). [496] Such dexamethasone-cyclophosphamide pulses were administered once a month and between these pulses the patient received 50 mg of cyclophosphamide orally daily. This regimen was referred as very effective in five patients with pemphigus vulgaris. After having administered a total of 14 to 48 dexamethasone-cyclophosphamide pulses, further treatment was withdrawn, followed by several years' remission. [507] A large study of 79 patients confirmed the good efficacy and safety of dexamethasone-cyclophosphamide pulses therapy. [508] The pulsed-cyclophosphamide regimen can be considered in severe or recalcitrant cases of pemphigus vulgaris.

The efficacy and safety of cyclophosphamide, azathioprine and cyclosporine as adjuvant drugs was evaluated and compared in 101 patients with pemphigus vulgaris. All therapy regimens had a similar safety profile preferring efficacy in cyclophosphamide. [509] Taken together, cyclophosphamide should be considered as an adjuvant drug of choice in the second line of treatment in moderate to severe pemphigus vulgaris.

Methotrexate

Methotrexate's primary metabolite polyglutamate competitively inhibits dihydrofolate reductase, preventing the reduction of folate cofactors. The metabolic disturbances result in the inhibition of purines and pyrimidines synthesis. Primarily, methotrexate was developed for the treatment of malignancies; subsequently its anti-inflammatory and immunosuppressive efficacy is utilized in the treatment of autoimmune disorders. In dermatology, methotrexate is most frequently used to treat psoriasis and T cell lymphoma. [510] It has been used for many other dermatologic conditions, including atopic dermatitis, vasculitides and bullous diseases, including pemphigus vulgaris. Methotrexate was the first adjuvant drug to be combined with corticosteroid in the management of pemphigus vulgaris. In the late 1960s and early 1970s, high doses of methotrexate were administered with high doses of prednisolone. Primarily, a methotrexate dose of 25-50 mg weekly or more up to 150 mg weekly was administered intramuscularly. [511] The combined therapy regimen was associated with very severe toxic effects, including the death of patients. [512] Accordingly, the use of methotrexate lost favor for the next 20-25 years. The use of methotrexate has recovered over the past two decades, following changes to the treatment regimen. At present, a dose of 10-20 mg of methotrexate is administered orally as a single dose each week. [481] The patient should be counseled to take the medication several hours before bedtime to help mask the fatigue and nausea. [512] Folic acid is used to decrease the deleterious side effects of methotrexate and can be used from 1 to 5 mg daily. Folic acid supplementation can prevent folate deficiency, improving tolerance and preventing anemia, neutropenia, stomatitis and oral ulcers. [512] In a methotrexate adverse event, the dose can escalate greater than 15 mg weekly. [511]

One analysis reported 136 patients with pemphigus vulgaris (from seven published studies) treated with methotrexate, among them 82% of patients showed clinical improvement, including 14 patients who were off all therapy at the end of evaluated period. Some clinical improvement was found in 13% of patients and all of them were considered to be methotrexate non-responders. [510] The cutaneous lesions respond usually very well to methotrexate therapy, but oral lesions have delayed healing. [511] Another study referred to clinical improvement in 91% of patients with pemphigus vulgaris. Seventy percent of patients were weaned off prednisolone completely, with a mean time to discontinuation of 18 months. [513] A limitation of this study was the small number of patients (23 patients). Another study showed a 50% reduction of systemic prednisolone after methotrexate therapy. [514] In the other study, systemic prednisolone was discontinued after 6 months of methotrexate therapy in six out of nine patients. [515]

The adverse effects of methotrexate are usually mild and self-limiting or preventable. However, in some cases they can be more severe. When adverse events occur, the dosage should be decreased or withdrawn. In a relatively short time, the adverse effects may consolidate in a normal condition. The most frequent adverse effects such as nausea, anorexia, vomiting, diarrhea, fatigue and malaise usually appear around initiation of therapy. [512] In general, these adverse events are dose dependent and may be minimized by taking the drug several hours before bedtime and by folic acid supplementation. One of the most serious adverse events is vicious myelosuppression, which can develop in patients assessing potential risk factors such as renal insufficiency, older age, concomitant illness or infections, hypoalbuminemia, drug overdose or drug interaction. [516] Medications that affect the folic acid pathway can be one of the serious sources of methotrexate toxicity. Sulfonamides and trimethoprim and some antibiotics may cause an important interaction with methotrexate, causing pancytopenia. [517] In addition, nonsteroidal anti-inflammatory drugs may interact with methotrexate, resulting in impaired renal clearance of methotrexate and significant toxicity. [518] In a 22-year long-term study of 157 psoriatic patients, myelosupression occurred in 10-20% of them, manifesting as macrocytic anemia, leucopenia, thrombocytopenia or pancytopenia. [519] In severe cases, myeolosuppression is considered a potentially fatal condition, but usually improves after dose reduction or the withdrawal of methotrexate. Patients with significant pancytopenia (WB <3000, Hg<11, platelets <50,000) should be treated immediately with leucovurin (folinic acid), the antidote to methotrexate that is able to bypass dihydrofolate reductase. [520] Folinic acid, in contrast to folic acid, does not require processing by dihydrofolate reductase for activity. Intravenous administration rapidly reverses acute methotrexate toxicity of bone marrow. Hepatotoxicity, including fibrosis and cirrhosis, is associated with long-term administration of methotrexate. According to the Manchester protocol, serum procolagen III aminopeptide (PIIINP)[13] assays may be used for monitoring liver toxicity produced by methotrexate. [521] This method can minimize the necessity for a liver biopsy to confirm liver damage and so methotrexate would become a more acceptable option for long-term administration. The limitation of this assay is the fact that the PIIINP level can be elevated in inflammatory conditions other than continuing hepatic fibrosis, and the assay is not currently readily available at many centers.

Methotrexate may cause reproductive toxicity. Pregnancy and lactation are both absolute contraindications because methotrexate is both abortifacient and teratogenic. [522, 523] Its small amount is also secreted in breast milk, with the effects on infants unknown. Because of methotrexate´s immunosuppressive properties, patients should be screened for evidence of any active infection prior to initiation of therapy. In several studies, low dose methotrexate reactivated a hepatitis B virus infection, and tuberculosis. [524, 525] If infection occurs, it should be appropriately treated. Mucocutaneous toxicity occurs more commonly in patients without adequate folic acid supplementation and in severe cases it could be associated with diarrhea and bone marrow toxicity. Mucositis and oral ulceration are not uncommon and may appear at any time in the course of treatment, being very painful. [526] In addition, mucous toxicity affects diet, causing weight loss resulting in a general deterioration of health. More rarely, ulceration in the skin has been reported, which could be an early harbinger of methotrexate toxicity. [527]

According to available data, methotrexate may be considered as second line treatment in the management of moderate to severe pemphigus vulgaris in patients whose disease is corticosteroid dependent, and in patients who develop significant complications to therapy. Once control over the initial disease is achieved using high doses of systemic corticosteroid, methotrexate may be used to maintain control of the disease, while allowing a reduction in the dose. According to this, methotrexate is considered a corticosteroid-sparing agent.

---

[13] PIIINP, procolagen III aminopeptide, is a metabolite of the formation of type III collagen. Its level becomes elevated in the serum as a damaged liver becomes fibrotic.

Cyclosporine

Cyclosporine is the first immunosuppressive drug allowing the regulating of T cells without excessive toxicity. Primarily, it was used after allogenic organ transplantation to reduce the risk of organ rejection. Cyclosporine is considered a calcineurin inhibitor, which in normal circumstances is responsible for activating the transcription of IL-2. In addition, it inhibits the production and release of IL-2, which leads to reduced function of effector T cells. Initial reports have referred that cyclosporine is an effective adjuvant drug with corticosteroid-sparing effect in pemphigus vulgaris. [528, 529, 530] A limitation of these studies was the small number of patients. In addition, the most important drawback of cyclosporine is the occurronce of clinically silent renal dysfunction, hypertension, tremor, hirsutism, and gingival hyperplasia, which may occur during long-term therapy. However, the other study compared the effectiveness and adverse effects of corticosteroid alone and a combination of corticosteroid and cyclosporine. The authors declared that combination treatment with corticosteroid and cyclosporine offers no advantage over treatment with just corticosteroid in patients with pemphigus vulgaris. In addition, complications were more common in patients who received combination therapy. [479] Taken together, the data are insufficient to support cyclosporine use in pemphigus vulgaris.

Tetracycline and Nicotinamide

Tetracyclines have anti-inflammatory and probably immunosuppressive properties. [531] The mechanism is not fully understood. Nicotinamide, the amide derivative of vitamin B_3, has been shown to exert anti-inflammatory properties by modulation of cytokine productions from immune cells, inhibition of lymphocyte blast formation and suppression of T cells. [532] The combination of tetracycline and nicotinamide has been used in the treatment of bullous pemphigoid, and linear IgA dermatosis. [533, 534] All these series documented the good efficacy of tetracycline and nicotinamide that have been used without another immunosuppressant.

In pemphigus vulgaris, medication consisting of tetracycline and niacinamide proved to be effective and corticosteroid-sparing in 51 patients with pemphigus (43 with pemphigus vulgaris and 8 with pemphigus foliaceus), corresponding with decreases in PV antibody levels with clinical improvement. [535] The safety profile was acceptable. [536] The limitation of most of the studies was the small number of patients with pemphigus vulgaris. Tetracyclines with or without nicotinamide could be considered as an adjuvant therapy in pemphigus, in several cases of mild pemphigus vulgaris.

Dapsone

Dapsone is a synthetic sulfone, aniline derivate that primarily possesses both antimicrobial and antiprotozoal activities. Additionally, dapsone has anti-inflammatory properties similar to non-steroidal anti-inflammatory drugs. [537] Recently, biologically active dapsone analogues like sulfoximine showed anti-cancer activity. [538] Numerous studies were conducted to discover the anti-inflammatory activity of dapsone in animal models, especially in small animals like mice, rats and guinea pigs, and in vitro models. Dapsone revealed inhibition of the reactive oxygen pathway, adhesion molecules activity, leukocytes chemotaxis, prostaglandins, leukotriens and IL-8, TNF-α, and others. [537] In pemphigus vulgaris, the anti-inflammatory activity of dapsone is used. Dapsone showed clinical improvement of pemphigus vulgaris controlled with a reduced level of PV antibodies. [539, 540] In another study, the authors speculated that the anti-inflammatory effect of dapsone may prove valuable in patients for whom corticosteroids are contraindicated or who develop significant side effects during long-term corticosteroid therapy. [505] The limitation of studies about dapsone is in their small number of patients. Because of lack of experiences, there is a little evidence to recommend dapsone in PV regimen.

Gold

In the past, several studies referred to the good efficacy of chrysotherapy in the treatment of moderate pemphigus vulgaris. The introduction of adjuvant modalities in pemphigus vulgaris repressed gold therapy. In recent times, new reports rediscovered gold efficacy in pemphigus vulgaris. The mechanism of gold activity has not been established, while it is recognized that it has an immunomodulatory efficacy in inflammatory diseases such as rheumatoid arthritis. [541]

The majority of data are confined to case reports and a small case series including pemphigus vulgaris cases of variable severity with short follow-up periods. One study referred about the good efficacy of gold intramuscular therapy in 62% (16/26) of patients with pemphigus vulgaris. [542] Another study reported that in 53.4% (7/13) of patients with pemphigus vulgaris, the use of gold resulted in complete clearing of the disease, discontinuation of all systemic therapies with long-term clinical remission. An improvement of pemphigus vulgaris allowed the gold dose to be reduced in remaining patients. [543] Two case reports demonstrated a clinical improvement of mucosal recalcitrant lesions in the oral cavity in pemphigus vulgaris patients treated with gold. [544]

Usually, treatment is started with an initial test dose of 10 mg followed by a 25 mg dose 1 week later, and subsequent 50 mg of intramuscular gold sodium thiomalate or aurothioglucose is administered weekly. [543] Adverse side effects including pruritus, allergic reaction, nausea, renal toxicity, and bone marrow suppression, are frequent, up to 42% and mostly reversible. [543] Aurofolin, an oral gold variant, seems to be associated with fewer and milder toxic effects. [542]

Taking together, gold is an adjuvant steroid-sparing agent that could be considered as an alternative to more established adjuvant drugs if they cannot be used.

Plasmapheresis

Plasmapheresis is more than a 20-year[14] old technique of plasma exchange used in the treatment of autoimmune diseases in which circulating autoantibodies are present, including pemphigus vulgaris. [545] The goal of plasmapheresis is to remove pathogenic

---

[14] Plasmapheresis was introduced in the treatment of pemphigus in 1978.

autoantibodies. The method consists of a procedure in which blood is drawn from the patient and a cell separator isolates the plasma. Subsequently, proteins are removed from the plasma, an appropriate substitute is added, and the composite is re-infused. [546] Plasmapheresis can be performed by a small or large volume exchange of plasma. A small-volume exchange consists of 400 ml of plasma substituted by equal volumes of saline or by 200 ml of 5% human albumin. This procedure is performed one to three times a week. Another treatment of choice is large-volume exchange. The last one is more effective in the case of pemphigus vulgaris. One plasma volume consists of 40-60 ml/kg body weight; the procedure can be repeated one to three times a week. [547] The regimen may consist of one or two large-volume plasmapheresis performed per month for 5-73 months. [548, 549] Long-term plasmapheresis demonstrated a clinical improvement in pemphigus vulgaris and has a considerable corticosteroid-sparing effect. [549]

Plasmapheresis is considered a relatively safe procedure. It can be associated with mild side effects, including hypotension, malaise, and fever in about 10-20% of patients. [547] Severe complications are rare and include infection and thrombosis of punctured veins, citrate toxicity, pulmonary edema, cardiac arrhythmias or anaphylactic reactions to foreign proteins. [550] Plasmapheresis is used in combination with corticosteroids in the treatment of corticosteroid-resistant pemphigus vulgaris. [549] The administration of just plasmapheresis without other medication is regularly associated with a rebound phenomenon[15]. The immediate rebound phenomenon can be prevented with a course of plasmapheresis within a relatively short period of time, e.g., five procedures of plasmapheresis in 10 days. The late rebound phenomenon is due to a negative feedback mechanism that stimulates an eruption of new autoantibody production by B cells in response to the rapid depletion of autoantibodies after the procedure. [548] The latter can be expected about 14 days after the first procedure and the antibody level can be ultimately higher than before plasmapheresis. [549] Administration of an immunosuppressant may inhibit the production of new autoantibodies. The timing of administration plays a crucial role in this procedure. Immunosuppressants' inhibitory effect on antibody rebound is most effective when given immediately after a course of plasmapheresis.

Various regimens can be used, including intravenous cyclophosphamide pulse therapy, intravenous prednisolone or other oral immunosuppressants such as azathioprine, mycophenolate mofetil and methotrexate. [550] In one study, 8 patients resistant to the conventional treatment regimen were treated with long-term plasmapheresis; all patients achieved a very good clinical improvement and long-time remission and revealed a corticosteroid-sparing effect. [549] The corticosteroid-sparing effect was also documented in plasmapheresis combined with dexamethasone or cyclophosphamide pulse therapy. [550] The other study compared two groups of patients with pemphigus vulgaris, each of 22 individuals; the first group was treated by prednisolone alone and the second group by prednisolone plus 10 large-volume plasmapheresis. The number of patients controlled at each therapeutic step did not differ between the two groups. Four deaths from sepsis were documented in the plasmapheresis group. [551]

---

[15] Rebound phenomenon in pemphigus presents with an increase of autoantibody titers following plasmapheresis within the first 3 hours after the procedure, due to passive re-diffusion of extracellular IgG back into the circulation. It can be replaced by about 50% of the IgG that has been removed.

Plasmapheresis cannot be recommended as a first-line therapy in patients with pemphigus vulgaris; it should instead be considered as a second-line treatment in recalcitrant pemphigus vulgaris not responding to conventional immunosuppressive regimens.

Immunoadsorption

Immunoadsorption, also termed immunoapheresis, is a more specific method than that of plasmapheresis. Immunoadsorption has a high affinity and selectivity in the removal of pathogenic autoantibodies and circulating immune complexes. The selectivity of immunoadsorption is more advantageous than plasmapheresis because plasmapheresis removes protective immunoglobulins, albumin and clotting factors, while immunoadsorption does not.

Immunoadsorption is associated with less essential plasma component loss; it does not have replacement protein infusion risks; allows the processing of the two to three-fold plasma volume per treatment session; and is associated with a lower rate of adverse events, such as infections and allergic reactions. [552] The first models used a genetically engineered antigen (Dsg) that represents the proper conformation of desmoglein antigen and contained most or all of the pathogenic epitopes. For this procedure, baculovirus vectors were used, expressing the entire extracellular domain of desmoglein antigen in eukaryotic cells. These proteins contained epitopes that all sera from patients with pemphigus vulgaris could be recognized. [553]

Nowadays, immunoadsorption systems use high-affinity adsorbers or low-affinity columns, and differ with respect to ligands, matrix, volume of columns, affinity to certain immunoglobulin classes and reusability. Autoantibody levels can be decreased by about 75% by a single procedure with a reusable system (Immunosorba and Therasorb), and after three procedures on three consecutive days (one cycle), autoantibody levels can be lowered by about 95%. [554] A single procedure is less effective because of rebound phenomenon from autoantibodies re-diffuse from the tissue to the circulation, which occurs 24 h after the procedure and 40% of the initial levels are reached again. [554] The Globaffin[16] adsorber system reduced the autoantibody level by an average of 50-70% per immunoadsorption cycle. [555] In contrast, other data indicate that the tryptophan adsorber achieved a 30% reduction. [556] Protein A adsorber [17] was evaluated as a rational, effective and safe adjuvant therapy. [557, 558] Clinically, mucosal and cutaneous improvements were documented in all protocols allowing for a reduction of systemic corticosteroids. In literature, all the data about the efficacy and safety of immunoadsorption are based on case series and case reports, accounting together 82 patients with pemphigus, among them 76 with pemphigus vulgaris. [559] In most patients, reusable systems on the basis of protein A were applied followed by a Globaffin adsorber column and then Therasorb[18] adsorber system. However, the factual value of immunoadsorption in pemphigus vulgaris is difficult to assess because no prospective

---

[16] Globaffin adsorber system contains GAM columns made with synthetic peptide GAM146.

[17] Protein A column contains *Staphylococcus aureus* protein A, which is covalently bounded to agarose-coupled beads. Protein A is a component of cellular wall of *S.aureus* and binds to the Fc portion of immunoglobulins or immune complexes.

[18] The Therasorb system contains immunoglobulin-columns coated with sheep immunoglobulins directed against human immunoglobulins.

controlled studies have yet been performed. Based on data from the studies, the efficacy of the immunoadsorption procedure in pemphigus vulgaris seems to rely on the rapid induction of clinical remission by a swift reduction in circulating autoantibodies during the first weeks of treatment, rather than the influence of long-term outcome. Any protocol is confirmed by authorities, but several protocols are used. Adjuvant immunosuppresion is obligatory and tapering doses of prednisolone combined with other adjuvant immunosuppressants such as azathioprine or mycophenolate mofetil are a standard regimen. Adverse events are relatively rare, documented with approximately <1 % of all procedures; among them are hypotension, deep venous thrombosis and sepsis. [560]

Taken together, the removal of pathogenic autoantibodies in pemphigus vulgaris by immunoadsorption is a rationale therapeutic approach that leads to rapid clinical responses and could be used to treat recalcitrant cases of pemphigus vulgaris where there has been failure to improve with more conventional therapies. To enhance the therapeutic effect with a durable remission, immunoadsorption may be applied in combination with the B cell depleting agent rituximab. In addition, prospective controlled trials are needed to fully appreciate immunoadsorption in the therapy regimen of pemphigus vulgaris.

Intravenous immunoglobulin

Intravenous immunoglobulin (IVIg) are a purified human source of the polyclonal immunoglobulin G (IgG) fraction extracted from pooled human plasma, via whole blood donors or by plasmapheresis. Both polyreactive natural antibodies and antibodies with specificities for allotypic antigens are present in the pool. [561] It has been suggested that these sources of immunoglobulin G contribute to IVIg efficacy through neutralization of various inflammatory components, including pathogenic antibodies, complements and Fas. [561]

Since IVIg's introduction in 1980 in intravenous form, IVIg has been used as replacement therapy in patients with primary and secondary immune deficiency and for treating autoimmune or inflammatory diseases. [562] In dermatology, IVIg is used mainly in the treatment of autoimmune disease and toxic epidermal necrolysis.

IVIG preparations belong to biologic treatments that are obtained from the pooled human plasma of between 3,000 and approximately 10,000 individual donors. [563] Clinical preparations of IVIg consist of intact IgG with the distribution of IgG subclasses corresponding to that of normal human serum, and probably contain a sampling from the entire repertoire of antigen-combining variable regions of antibodies that would be present in normal serum. Commercially prepared IVIg preparations are not identical and refer to the naturally occurring autoantibodies as found in normal serum. The large number of donors in the pool naturally increases the risk of diluting any rare specific activity and the risk of transmission of latent infections. All manufactures providing production of human plasma must adhere to guidelines when obtaining and processing plasma to ensure product safety. National authorities are responsible for authorizing the preparations. The half-time of IVIg in normal individual is approximately 3 weeks.

The mechanism of IVIG possesses a complex of various activities that are not fully understood in vivo. Several mechanisms are proposed to act either individually or in combination in the following pathways. The first of the pathways comprises the immunomodulatory role of anti-idiotypic antibodies that regulate the autoreactive repertoires by neutralizing autoantibodies. IVIg contains anti-idiotypes against a number of disease-associated autoantibodies, including those against factor VIII, thyroglobulin, DNA, intrinsic factor, peripheral-nerve gangliosides, platelet gpIIb/IIIa, the acetylcholine receptor, endothelial cells, phospholipids, nephritic factor and retinal autoantigens-β. [564] Anti-idiotypic antibodies are effective in the treatment or prevention of disease because they inhibit the binding of the pathogenic autoantibodies to their corresponding antigen. In addition, IVIg may act via the idiotypic network, causing soluble circulating immune complexes to aggregate and become insoluble and consequently, removable by the reticuloendothelial system. [565] The efficacy of IVIg in the prevention of blistering formations was demonstrated in an experimental pemphigus vulgaris model. [566] The other study referred that anti-desmoglein-specific IVIg is more effective than regular IVIg in the same pemphigus vulgaris model. [565] The last model utilized the Dsg-specific IVIg that was affinity-purified from IVIg on a column of single-chain variable fragment anti-Dsg1 and anti-Dsg3 IVIg.

The other activity is that of the immunomodulatory effect of the F_C[19] fragment region of the IgG that allows interactions and signal transductions by $F_{C\gamma}$ receptors on numerous immune cells. [563] These immunomodulatory effects of IVIg are probably mediated by the interactions between IgG and both high-affinity $F_{C\gamma}RI$ and low-affinity $F_{C\gamma}RII$ and $F_{C\gamma}RIII$ receptors in immune competent cells (monocytes, macrophages, dendritic cells). [564] However, IVIg might also modulate the expression or affinity of these receptors and saturate the $F_{C\gamma}R$, additionally monomeric IgG in IVIg contains antagonist of human $F_{C\gamma}RII$ and $F_{C\gamma}RIII$ and decreases $F_{C\gamma}RIIA$ on dendritic cells. [567-569] Among several mechanisms explaining the mode of IVIg activity, some lines of evidence have suggested that the neonatal Fc receptor for IgG (FcRn)[20] plays an important role for rapid clearance of pathogenic antibodies in pemphigus vulgaris. [570] In the mouse model, directly implicated FcRn blockade was confirmed as a significant mechanism of IVIg anti-inflammatory action. [571] These results suggest that saturation of the FcRn results in the accelerated clearance of IgG and so a reduction in the levels of pathogenic antibodies. Other IVIg activity is that of the anti-complement mechanism. IVIg binds the activated complements C3b and C4b in a C1q-independent and C1q-dependent fashion, thus preventing the deposition of these fragments on target surfaces of complement activation. [571] IVIg modulates the production of cytokines and cytokine antagonists. This activity is considered to be the major *in vivo* mechanism by which IVIg exerts its anti-inflammatory effect. [561] IVIg modulates Th1 and Th2 cytokine production. [564] IVIg was also found to selectively induce gene transcription and the secretion of IL-1receptor antagonist (IL-1ra) and IL-8 in cultures of normal human monocytes that were enhanced in the presence of autologous T cells. [572] Among these activities, IVIg increases the level of inhibitors of apoptotic proteins (IAPs) that can target the caspases, and increases in their level lead to resistance of apoptosis. [573] The anti-apoptotic effect of IVIg on keratinocytes is well known in toxic epidermal necrolysis. [574] In addition, IVIg interacts with a number of membrane molecules on T cells, B cells and monocytes relevant to control

---

[19] Fc regions of IgG allow antibodies to interact with Fc γ receptors (Fc$_{C\gamma}$R) on phagocytes. Fab regions recognize the antigenic target and provide diversity to antibodies.

[20] FcRn is the MHC class I family-like receptors, are normally responsible for extending the life span of serum IgG antibodies. Whether this molecule contributes to autoimmune pathogenesis remains unclear.

their autoreactivity and to induce their tolerance to self-tissue. Interaction between IVIg and idiotypes of receptors on B cell provide the basis for the ability of IVIg to regulate autoreactive B cell clones *in vivo*. [575] IVIg also inhibits the differentiation and maturation of dendritic cells *in vitro* and abrogates the capacity of mature dendritic cells to secrete IL-12 on activation while enhancing IL-10 production. IVIg induces down-regulation of co-stimulatory molecules associated with modulation of cytokine secretion that results in inhibition of autoreactive and alloreactive Tcell activation and proliferation. [576]

Diagnostic criteria for the use of IVIG therapy include the failure of conventional therapy, significant adverse effects of conventional therapy, contraindications to the use of high dose long-term systemic or adjuvant therapies, progressive disease that is uncontrolled, rapid, and debilitating. [577] A response to IVIg should be demonstrated on review at 6 months. If there is no response to treatment after 6 cycles of treatment, discontinuation of the IVIg treatment is advisable. Adjuvant therapy with IVIg should be administered every 4 weeks initially. If the clinical response is good, the interval between infusions can be increased gradually to a maximum of 6 weeks. The recommended total dose of 2 g/kg by infusion is used to treat autoimmune bullous disorders, including pemphigus vulgaris. Treatment should be administered over a period of 3-5 consecutive days, with fractionated administration of the IVIg therapy contributing to better tolerability. For evidence based on economic reasons, the IVIg is recommended as second-line treatment in pemphigus vulgaris. However, contraindications to standard immunosuppressive therapy like aseptic bone necrosis, poorly controlled diabetes, advanced osteoporosis and cataracts, may in individual cases qualify the use of IVIg as a first-line treatment. Nevertheless, IVIg should only be used as a second-line treatment in combination with corticosteroids and another immunosuppressive agent. Generally, monotherapy with IVIg is not recommended. IVIg may be beneficial in patients who do not have a response to standard therapies or who experience serious side effects from systemic corticosteroids or adjuvant therapies. Follow-up criteria assess clinical improvement, decreased titres of serum anti-Dsg antibodies, whether systemic corticosteroids can be gradually discontinued, total dose and duration of therapy, and the number of relapses before and after the initiation of IVIg therapy.

Until 2009, only case reports and small uncontrolled studies analyzing IVIg in pemphigus vulgaris have been reported. Recent reports on the efficacy of IVIg in pemphigus vulgaris identified up to 150 patients with pemphigus treated with IVIg in case series. [577] About 90% of these patients responded to IVIg when given in conjunction with systemic corticosteroids with or without adjuvant agents. The clinical improvement of IVIG was usually rapid and associated with a decline in serum autoantibodies. [578] Effective clinical control was most frequently achieved after 4 to 6 months. In 2009, the first multicentre randomized placebo-controlled double-blind trial conducted on 61 patients with pemphigus treated them with a single cycle of cumulative IVIg 2 g, 1 g or 0 divided into 5 consecutive days (reported as 400 mg, 200 mg, 0 mg daily). The study documented a significantly higher efficacy in 2 g dose regimen compared to those of 1 g and placebo. A decrease of autoantibody level (ELISA) lined the clinical improvement of pemphigus and the good safety profile of IVIg was confirmed in both treated groups. [579] There are several studies about the corticosteroid-sparing effect of IVIg. [580-582] In one case series study, the effect of IVIG was evaluated in 10 patients with severe recalcitrant pemphigus vulgaris using PDAI evaluating score. After the first IVIG cycle, the PDAI score decreased by an average of 36.5%, while after the second IVIG cycle and after the third IVIG cycle the PDAI score decreased by 48.5% and 73%. Six months after IVIG treatment, the PDAI had decreased by 91% of the baseline value. The clinical improvement followed the titre of PV antibody. The corticosteroid-sparing effect was documented with a decrease of 38%, 69% and 88% after the first, second and third IVIG cycles, respectively, with a 92% decrease achieved after 6 months follow-up. The immunomodulation effect with long-lasting efficacy was achieved in all patients, while none of them revealed a relapse of disease after two years follow-up and one patient was off therapy. [583] Another study of 20 patients with pemphigus vulgaris documented a higher decrease in PV antibody levels when IVIG was co-administered with cytotoxic drugs. [584] In addition, the safety of IVIg was confirmed in one case series of eight pregnant patients with active pemphigus vulgaris. No long-term adverse effects of IVIg were observed in either the mother or the child based on a long-term follow-up. [585] IVIg was also referred as a drug with good safety profile in eight patients with juvenile pemphigus vulgaris. [586]

Adverse effects are usually mild and self-limited. The incidence of adverse effects of IVIg in patients treated for autoimmune disease is usually lower than 1%. [493] Another study documented no serious adverse event. Headache (43.8%) and fatigue (43.8%) were the most common side effects in one case series study of 16 patients with autoimmune bullous disorders. [587] Systemic adverse reactions can be immediate (60% of all reactions) occurring within 6 hours of an infusion. A delayed reaction (40% of all reactions) occurs within 6 hours to one week after infusion, and late reaction (less than 1% of reactions), occurring weeks and months after infusion. [588] Immediate systemic reactions include headache and other body aches, chills and fever. Immediate anaphylactic and anaphylactoid reactions are uncommon. The most common delayed systemic reaction is persistent headache. Less common but more serious delayed reactions include aseptic meningitis, renal failure, thromboebolism, and hemolytic reactions. Late reactions are uncommon, but often severe, including lung disease, enteritis and infectious diseases.

Immediate serious adverse events include anaphylaxis, which can develop in patients with IgA deficiency, because some preparation may contain a trace of IgA. [589] Another serious adverse effect is aseptic meningitis. The onset of this event is usually within 6 to 24 hours from infusion. Patients with a history of migraine headaches are more susceptible to this condition. [590] However, the risk of thromboembolic event was demonstrated as uncommon despite the presence of risk factors. [591] To minimize adverse events it is recommended to limit the daily IVIg dose to 400-500 mg/kg, to consider pre- and post-infusion hydratation, and to use a slow infusion rate (e.g., 50 mg/kg for the first hour then 100 mg/kg/hour). A high infusion rate and high doses have been identified as potential risk factors for adverse effects. Pregnancy is not a contraindication for IVIg therapy. [493]

Taken together, IVIg is a very effective therapy in pemphigus vulgaris and has a very good safety profile. It is recommended as a second-line therapy to treat moderate to severe pemphigus vulgaris. However, the use of IVIG is limited because therapy is expensive and penalizes patients and their widespread use.

Rituximab

Rituximab, is a human/murine chimeric antibody that specifically targets the trans-membrane protein CD20 of B cells. This CD20 antigen is not expressed by plasma cells, stem cells, or B cell progenitors. Rituximab induced B cell depletion resulted in a significant improvement of morbidity in many autoimmune diseases, including pemphigus vulgaris. Primarily, rituximab was used for treating non-Hodgkin´s B cell lymphoma. The use of rituximab in pemphigus began after a marked improvement in lymphoma-associated autoimmune phenomena, such as paraneoplastic pemphigus. [592]

Rituximab activity is a complex of multiple mechanisms resulting in B cell depletion. These effector mechanisms may act individually or in combination to deplete B cells, depending on disease pathology. [593] After the binding of rituximab to its cell-surface receptor, $CD4^+$ B cells are killed by a combination of antibody-dependent cellular cytotoxicity by natural killer (NK) cells, complement-dependent toxicity, and apoptosis, and remain absent from circulation for 6 to 12 months. Differential susceptibility of malignant and autoreactive B cells to rituximab may depend on the expression of complement regulatory molecules such as CD46, CD55 and CD59 on the target cells. [594] Opsonization of B cells by rituximab may also help to induce the clearance of B cells in circulation through phagocytosis by the reticuloendothelial system. [595] The reticuloendothelial system also acts in the clearance of apoptotic B cells after rituximab therapy. However, complement mediated B cell depletion is considered to be the main mechanism involved in the rituximab effect on malignant B cells. [596] Complement mediated effects are fast acting. Conversely, removing or killing rituximab opsonized B cells by NK cells or macrophages may take longer since these cells have to be recruited and must interact with opsonized B cells for their function. Apoptosis induced by rituximab cross linking of CD20 on B cells may also be an effective mechanism for B cell depletion. [596] However, after rituximab treatment, B cell counts returned to normal levels, but autoimmune disease did not relapse in a significant number of patients. These data suggest that rituximab mediated B cell depletion may have a positive influence on other cells of the immune system and may contribute to the re-establishment of immune tolerance and homeostasis. One study documented that rituximab-mediated depletion of B cells resulted in the generation of $FoxP3^+$Treg cells, along with down regulation of CD40 expression. [597] Treg cells are effective suppressors of autoimmune responses in autoimmune diseases, including pemphigus vulgaris. However, B cells require T cell help to produce antibodies through CD40-CD40 L interactions. Down regulation of CD40-CD40L interactions may participate in the re-establishment of immune tolerance by down regulating T cell help to B cells during the re-population of the B cell compartment after rituximab therapy. [596, 598] The effect of rituximab on the clinical course of the disease can only be determined if a significant long-term follow-up is provided. It is important to know the time at which the B cells repopulate to a normal level. It was documented that B cell depletion persists for 6-12 months; however, 3 years B cell depletion was also referred. [599] Some patients may not achieve a B cell recovery for 18-24 months and during this period are susceptible to infection. [596] Furthermore, the recovery to normal levels of B cells can be delayed in elderly patients. Prolonged immunosuppresion has been associated with increased incidence of cancer. It is well known that rituximab has a late onset of action and in order to control early disease activity it needs to be combined with corticosteroids and/or adjuvant agents.

There are two FDA approved protocols for rituximab treatment in pemphigus. The first protocol uses two infusions at a dose of 1g of rituximab, given two weeks apart (lymphoma protocol); the second one utilizes four infusions of rituximab at a dose of 375 mg/m^2 given in four consecutive weeks, a week apart (rheumatoid arthritis protocol). However, the biological behavior of B cells in lymphoma patients is different from that of patients with pemphigus. The rheumatoid arthritis protocol could prove better because both rheumatoid arthritis and pemphigus are autoimmune diseases. However, the rheumatoid arthritis protocol utilizes BSA-dependent dosing, which is accompanied by possible dosing errors and a higher pharmacokinetic variability. [600]

Given the many practical advantages, fixed dosing is recommended to be the first option in the studies. The most recent strategy is to find a suitable and effective regimen with good risk rate to benefit. One cycle of treatment may be repeated. [601] The administered dose of rituximab should be infused intravenously over 4-5 hours. Premedication before each infusion is recommended with an antipyretic, e.g., paracetamol 1000 mg orally, as well as antihistamine. Prior to the first infusion, prednisolone 100 mg is also advised.

So far, no prospective controlled clinical trial on rituximab treatment for pemphigus vulgaris has been published. A recent review evaluated the efficacy of rituximab in more than 140 patients with pemphigus vulgaris derived from case reports and case series. Complete remission, clinical remission and partial remission were achieved in about 40%, 40% and 15% of patients, respectively. [577] In most patients, lesions started to heal within just a few weeks after the first rituximab infusion. A maximal effect was documented after 3 to 4 months. [602, 603] In another study, of 31 PV patients treated with rituximab, complete remission was achieved in 18 (58%) patients; with the median duration of remission at 19 to 21 months. Eight (44%) of 18 patients relapsed 6-17 months after treatment. The authors of this study suggest that patients treated with rituximab earlier in the course of the disease may have better outcomes. [604]

The rituximab mechanism of action supports the rationale for early therapy. It is well known that short-term rituximab therapy of severe pemphigus vulgaris appears to be safe and effective. Good efficacy was also confirmed over the long term. However, the long-term remission rate without therapy in the rituximab group (n=13) did not differ significantly from that of the control subject (n=11) treated with corticosteroids alone or in combination with an adjuvant agent. [605] Another retrospective study evaluated 47 patients treated biweekly with 1g of rituximab. Remission rates after the first treatment cycle reached 76%. Repeating treatment further increased the remission rates to 91%. The relapse rate was 22% at a median time of 8 months, but 75% of relapsing achieved remission again with additional cycles. Immediate post-infusion PV exacerbation was documented in 4 patients. [606] One case report also documented exacerbation immediately after the first rituximab infusion. Repeat rituximab infusions were administered 3 months after the first infusion in 3-monthly intervals, followed by total remission achieved 11 months after the first infusion; moreover, a drop in corticosteroids was documented. [606]

In light of the above observations, repeated infusion of rituximab ameliorates the remission rate in patients who failed with one cycle of rituximab. Actually, the post-infusion exacerbation cannot be explicated, as well as the long delayed efficacy of rituximab. A recent study evaluated a low-dose of rituximab in a single course of two infusions of rituximab (500 mg each) at an interval of 2 weeks as an effective and safe treatment in 15 patients with pemphigus. Relapses occurred, mostly at the end of the second year. [607] Another study documented an alternative dosing regimen as a single cycle of rituximab, 1g on day 1 and day 15 as an effective treatment for patients with pemphigus vulgaris. All 9 patients were concurrently treated with prednisolone, immunosuppressive agents and/or IVIg. All patients had a partial remission initially between 4 and 16 weeks after rituximab treatment. At the end of the observation period (a minimum of 6 months), 3 of 9 patients (33%) were in complete remission and 3 (33%) were in partial remission and 4 (44%) had a recurrence requiring a second cycle of rituximab. [608]

If an alternative regimen would be confirmed with a prospective control study, it could be more convenient for patients because it shortens the number of clinic visits to receive the infusion, as well as the cost of rituximab. Recently, a randomized, comparative, observer - blinded study of 22 patients with pemphigus evaluated 2 dose regimens, namely 1g on day 0 and 15 or 500 mg of rituximab. In this study, there was no statistical difference in the time taken to achieve any of primary end points between the two groups. The relapses were more common in patients who received low-dose rituximab, and the time to relapse was also earlier in patients on a low dose. An immunological evaluation showed a statistically significant decrease in anti-Dsg antibody levels only in the 1g regimen of rituximab. There was, however, no difference in the B cell depletion achieved between the two groups. [609] Taken together, the low dose of rituximab indicates inadequate B cell depletion leading to early and more frequent relapses.

Ahmed et al. referred about combination therapy of rituximab and IVIg that was used to treat 11 patients with refractory widespread and prolonged pemphigus vulgaris. All patients had limited or incomplete responses to conventional treatment, including IVIg alone. All of them had had numerous relapses and remissions associated with multiple side effects and hospitalizations. The induction therapy started with two cycles of rituximab once per week for 3 weeks and IVIg in the fourth week. After that, the protocol followed a monthly infusion of rituximab and IVIg for 4 consecutive months. Nine of 11 patients had a clinical remission lasting 22 to 37 months. The combination of rituximab and IVIg showed a high corticosteroid-sparing effect and additionally, all immunosuppressive therapy, including prednisolone, was discontinued before ending rituximab treatment in all 9 patients. Titres of PV antibodies correlated with disease activity. Peripheral blood B cells became undetectable shortly after initiating rituximab therapy, but subsequently returned to normal values. [603] In another study, the combination of rituximab and IVIg therapy documented a long-term remission in 58% (11/19) of patients, while 42% (8/19) of patients experienced relapses. The time to depletion, repopulation or return to pretreatment levels of B cells were similar in both groups of patients with long-term remission or with relapse. In relapsed patients, retreatment achieved long-term remission. Interestingly, in patients with mucocutaneous disease, PV antibody levels increased during clinical relapse. [610]

Shimanovich et al. showed a more vigorous reduction in serum PV antibody levels in the initial stage of treatment using a protocol of a combination of protein A immunoadsorption with rituximab and conventional immunosuppressants in patients with severe pemphigus vulgaris. Patients who failed to respond to this therapy subsequently received IVIg. The combination of protein A immunoadsorption and rituximab demonstrated both a rapid decline of circulating autoantibody levels and a rapid improvement of cutaneous and mucosal lesions within 4 weeks of therapy in four of seven patients. Three patients were resistant to rituximab and showed a good response to IVIg therapy. The long-term response of 13-30 months of follow-up showed one patient in complete remission without any immunosuppressive therapy. Another three patients are in complete remission on immunosuppressive therapy or in partial remission. The remaining three patients failed to show any long-term improvement on the protein A immunoadsorption and rituximab combination regimen. [611] The new treatment protocol could be effective in a subset of patients with severe refractory pemphigus vulgaris. Interestingly, approximately half of the patients (3/7) with severe pemphigus vulgaris were resistant to rituximab and had a good response to IVIg.

Serious adverse reactions occur in only a small minority of patients, but overall rituximab therapy is safe. The majority of patients receiving their first infusion of rituximab have experience with flu-like syndromes, nausea, headache, fatigue and rush. The most acute side effects of rituximab are mild, transient, and infusion-related. In immediate reactions, treatment should be discontinued. If possible, after waiting a half hour the rituximab infusion can be continued at a slow rate (half flow rate). Corticosteroids and antihistamines should be re-administered. [601] About 10% of patients develop more severe adverse effects, including bronchospasm, hypoxia and hypotension. [612] Rituximab must be stopped and supportive therapy administered as required, consisting of corticosteroids, oxygen, bronchodilators, and intravenous saline. Adverse events were markedly lower following the second treatment compared with the first one. [613] The use of paracetamol, antihistamines and corticosteroids is recommended as a pretreatment to help control infusion related reactions. [612] Rituximab associated infections are related to depletion of the B cell component of the immune system. Pooled data from 356 patients receiving rituximab showed 30% of patients with an infection; 19% of patients had bacterial infections, 10% viral infections and 1% of patients had fungal infections. Severe infections, including sepsis, occurred in 1% of patients during the treatment and 2% of patients during the follow-up period. [612] In a small series of 21 patients with pemphigus, two severe adverse effects were documented as following pyelonephritis as a delayed infection 12 months after rituximab therapy, and one patient died from septicemia 18 months after rituximab therapy. [602] Moreover, patients are frequently on concomitant immunosuppressive therapies, which also contribute to increased susceptibility to infections and in a certain group of patients may predispose the development of severe infections that can infrequently lead to death. Therefore, patients on multiple immunosuppressive drugs should be closely monitored for infectious complications. In autoimmune disease, including pemphigus vulgaris, significantly high titers of human anti-chimeric antibodies (HACA) against rituximab were associated with failure to deplete B cells. [614] However, the long-term consequences of rituximab therapy in patients with autoimmune disease, including pemphigus vulgaris, are unknown. Rituximab is contraindicated in pregnancy, children and adolescents. Finally, rituximab therapy appears to have a good risk to benefit ratio based on currently available data.

Taken together, treatment with rituximab resulted both in a major clinical improvement and corticosteroid-sparing effects. The current standard of care typically indicates rituximab for late treatment of pemphigus vulgaris as a second line therapy, after conventional treatments failed.

Topical Therapy

In pemphigus vulgaris, topical therapy is considered to be supplementary to systemic therapy. Above all, topical therapy is used to prevent or treat secondary infection, to stimulate the re-epithelization of denuded areas and to reduce pain.

Corticosteroids possess anti-inflammatory and anti-acantholytic activity in both systemic and topical administration. Topical treatment can be used supplementary to systemic treatment or as a sole treatment in localized disease. When topical corticosteroids are used on a limited surface area, they don't reveal systemic efficacy. Scattered case reports referred about their efficacy and good risk to benefit ratio in the treatment of autoimmune bullous pemphigoid. [615] This was the main motive to utilize them also in the management of pemphigus vulgaris. Only several case reports documented their efficacy and safety to treat pemphigus vulgaris. One study documented topical efficacy as a single therapy of seven patients with mild pemphigus vulgaris and pemphigus foliaceus. A very potent topical (clobetasol propionate) corticosteroid was used. In all patients the disease was controlled initially with healing of cutaneous lesions within 15 days, while the healing of mucosal lesions took at least 1 month. [616] The follow-up was very short because localized relapses occurred on previously involved areas soon after discontinuation of treatment. Another approach of topical corticosteroids is their use as an additive therapy to systemic corticosteroids or adjuvant agents. Topical corticosteroids may support systemic agents and advocate healing through their topical anti-inflammatory and anti-acantholytic activity. They are successfully used to treat solitary lesions in patients on maintenance therapy to control the disease. In addition, intralesional injection, e.g., tramcinolone acetonide, can be used in recalcitrant individual lesions to avoid enhancing the systemic immunosuppressive agent to control disease. However, a high dose may cause local and temporary atrophy of the skin. This adverse effect should be considered and evaluated both in terms of risk and benefit.

Recently, several case reports referred about topical administration of calcineurin inhibitors, namely tacrolimus and pimecrolimus. [616] Both are used in dermatology as an alternative therapy to topical corticosteroids with better safety profile, because they don´t cause atrophy. In all reports, both are used in combination with systemic immunosuppressive agents, mostly with corticosteroids. Both were utilized especially to treat recalcitrant solitary PV lesions with good efficacy. [617-620] A double -blind placebo-controlled trial evaluated the efficacy of pimecrolimus in the treatment of pemphigus vulgaris. The 11 patients with pemphigus vulgaris enrolled to the study manifested 62 cutaneous lesions. Pimecrolimus revealed a significantly higher epithelization index than the placebo. [621] Both should be a good alternative to topical corticosteroids.

Another new approach in topical treatment of pemphigus vulgaris is the epidermal growth factor (EGF) in cream. Firstly, the topical EGF was successfully used to treat diabetic foot and burn. [622, 623] Moreover, EGF innovative treatment helped re-epithelization of PV lesions and significantly reduced healing time. [624]

Another approach is nicotinamide used as an adjuvant systemic agent in PV regimens. Recently, nicotinamide gel was used to treat PV lesions in a double blind placebo controlled study in eight patients with a total of 60 skin lesions. After 30 days of treatment, the epithelization index in skin lesions that received nicotinamide was significantly higher than that of the placebo. [625]

Controlled comparative trials are needed to determine the place of calcineurin inhibitors, nicotinamide, and epidermal growth factor in topical treatment of pemphigus vulgaris. These new approaches may broaden the option of anti-inflammatory topical agents that may influence the autoimmune background of pemphigus vulgaris and aid treatment additionally with systemic immunosuppressive agents.

Generally, the skin lesions in pemphigus vulgaris should be protected against infections and cleaned using a physiological saline or diluted bacteriostatic solutions, e.g., potassium permanganate, silver nitrate or chlorhexidine. Long-term refractory solitary lesions that do not respond to immunosuppressive regimen should be cultured to exclude secondary infection such as candidiasis, herpes simplex or gram positive or gram negative bacterial infection, and be treated according to the cause and culture sensitivity. Pain and sticking of clothing can be reduced with a light coating of ointment such as vaseline.

Treatment of oral lesions is very difficult and their response to systemic agents, as well as topical agents, is much slower than those on the skin. The recommended administration is to use high-potency corticosteroids in an oral adherent base or to let tablets of corticosteroids dissolve in the oral cavity, better than swallowing, and rinsing with dexamethasone solution, can also be used. In addition, solitary recalcitrant lesions may respond to intralesional injection of triamcinolon acetonide at a concentration of 20µg/L. Topical anesthetics are recommended as further treatment.

The new approach to release the pain of PV lesions in the oral cavity is to use a concentrated oral gel containing polyvinylpyrrolidone and sodium hyaluronate (Gelclair). It forms an adherent barrier and layer covering of oral mucosa lesions, thus protecting sensitive nerve endings and lubricating and coating the damaged tissue. This preparation is mostly used in oncology in patients with oral mucositis after intensive chemotherapy or radiotherapy, as well as in conditions of various etiologies including oral surgery, traumatic ulcers caused by braces of ill-fitting dentures. It could also be used to protect painful lesions in the oral cavity in PV patients. Several studies documented its efficacy as follows: it decreased pain in the oral cavity and did not worsen oral bacterial and yeast colonization, and probably even helped to protect mucosa from *Enteroccocus* and *Candida sp.* in transplant patients with oral mucositis. [626, 627] Caphosol is the second oral mouthwash used to treat oral mucositis in cancer patients. Caphosol is an electrolyte solution, designed in part to replace the normal ionic pH balance in the oral cavity. When mixed together, the calcium solution and phosphate solution form a stable supersaturated calcium phosphate (Ca^{2+}/PO_4^{-3}) mouthwash with a composition resembling that of natural saliva. It has been supposed that this high ionic content may aid in tissue repair by diffusing ions into the intercellular spaces. [628] Contrary results documented efficacy in treating or preventing the oral mucositis and in reducing pain. [629-631] Despite these observation results in cancer patients, Caphosol may be useful in the management of oral lesions in pemphigus. Both mouth washes Gelclair and Caphosol should be evaluated in a pemphigus study.

Topical analgetics or anesthetics and antiseptic mouthwashes are recommended as further treatment. Various preparations contain lidocain in gel or oral rinse to decrease oral pain and potentially improve the ability to drink and eat in PV patients.

Oral hygiene requires attention because it seems that bacteria may aggravate both healing and also yeast infection. A gentle technique using a soft-bristle brush should be used to clean the teeth twice daily. Antiseptic mouthwashes should be used several times a day. Treatment of periodontal disease is important. Pain in the throat after swallowing should be assessed by endoscopic examination to distinguish whether it is due to recurrent PV disease or secondary candidiasis. Secondary yeast infection is a recurrent problem and should be recognized early and treated with antimycotic troches or systemically.

Taken together, corticosteroids alone or with corticosteroid-sparing immunosuppressive agents such as azathioprine and mycophenolate mofetil, remain the first-line treatment in pemphigus vulgaris. The second-line treatment consists of several corticosteroid-sparing agents such as cyclophosphamide, methotrexate and dapsone. The high incidence of side and adverse effects of corticosteroids shows the way to find new approaches in the management of pemphigus vulgaris. New approaches have progressed in recent years; therapeutic modalities have been extended by new drugs and interventions, which have changed the prognosis and outcome of pemphigus vulgaris. New modalities include IVIg, immunoadsorption and rituximab, which may be used as second-line therapy for patients with pemphigus vulgaris being refractory to conventional treatment. New regimens are looking for such as an alternative treatment or low-dose treatment in rituximab, which could have benefits for patients resulting in lower dose administration and a better safety profile. Prospective controlled studies have been initiated for new therapies, including IVIg, immunoadsorption, and rituximab. New approaches directed at inducing healing of solitary PV lesions in the maintenance phase without raising the dose of systemic immunosuppressive agent show new topical agents administered to skin lesions and also to mucosal lesions. Topical corticosteroids were confirmed to improve the healing of singular lesions in the maintenance phase of treatment. In recent years, new modalities are used that may augment or replace topical corticosteroids with better safety profile. The oral mucosa involvement is still a challenge, but new additional modalities from oncology may aid in healing mucosal lesions.

CONCLUSION

Hitherto, there is still no confirmed "best treatment strategy" for pemphigus. This may be due to the disease's rarity, to the fact that it has various phenotypes, and to its variable severity. However, the management of pemphigus must take into account the disease's impact on various aspects of the patient's life, including physical, emotional and functional involvement, which should be considered before deciding on the optimal therapeutic protocol. In the long list of immunosuppressants recommended for treatment of pemphigus, corticosteroids remain the mainstay despite their frequent and numerous side and adverse effects. Adjuvant drugs are usually administered in combination with systemic corticosteroids so as to reduce related side effects and increase the drug efficacy. Recently, adjuvant immunosuppressants and immunomodulators have been applied as initial treatment in combination with corticosteroids in order to decrease the initial dose of corticosteroids.

A new approach in pemphigus management is IVIg. It is a very effective therapy in pemphigus vulgaris and has a very good safety profile. It is recommended as a second-line therapy to treat moderate to severe pemphigus. Another new tool in pemphigus management is rituximab. The treatment with rituximab resulted both in a major clinical improvement and corticosteroid-sparing effects. The current standard of care typically indicates rituximab for late treatment of pemphigus vulgaris as a second line therapy, after conventional treatments failed.

Very important in management of pemphigus is the topical treatment. Generally, the skin lesions in pemphigus should be protected against infections and cleaned using a physiological saline or diluted bacteriostatic solutions. Treatment of oral lesions is very difficult and their response to systemic agents, as well as topical agents, is much slower than those on the skin. The new approach to release the pain of pemphigus lesions in the oral cavity is to use a concentrated oral gel containing polyvinylpyrrolidone and sodium hyaluronate (Gelclair). It forms an adherent barrier and layer covering of oral mucosa lesions, thus protecting sensitive nerve endings and lubricating and coating the damaged tissue. Caphosol is the second oral mouthwash that could be used to treat oral pemphigus lesions. Caphosol is an electrolyte solution, designed in part to replace the normal ionic pH balance in the oral cavity with a composition resembling that of natural saliva. It has been supposed that this high ionic content may aid in tissue repair by diffusing ions into the intercellular spaces. Both oral medications are successfully used in oncologic patients to treat oral mucositis after cytostatic therapy. Both might widen the list of oral medication used in pemphigus vulgaris.

Pemphigus is a rare disease and to find a correlation between various aspects implicated in the pathogenesis and treatment of the disease requires a large number of patients and this fact complicates the evaluation of previous and also future studies.

REFERENCES

[1]   Buc, M. 2014. *Basic and clinical immunology.* 3rd Edition. Comenius University, Bratislava, 126-140.

[2]   Hietanen, J., Salo, O.P. 1982. Pemphigus: an epidemiological study of patients treated in Finish hospitals between 1969 and 1978. *Acta Derm. Venereol.* 62, 491-96.

[3]   Pisanti, S., Sharay, Y., Kaufman, E., Posner, L.N. 1974. Pemphigus vulgaris: incidence in Jews of different ethnic groups, according to age, sex, and initial lesion. *Oral. Surg. Oral. Med. Oral. Pathol.* 38, 382-87.

[4]   Hans-Filho, G., dos Santos, V., Katayama, J.H., Aoki, V., Rivitti, E.A., Sampaio, S.A., Friedman, H., Moraes, J.R., Moraes, M.E., Eaton, D.P., Lopez, A.L., Hoffman, R.G., Fairley, J.A., Guidice, G.J., Diaz, L.A. 1996. An active focus of high prevalence of fogo selvagem on an Ameridian reservation in Brazil. Cooperative Group on Fogo Selvagem Research. *J. Invest. Dermatol.* 107, 68-75.

[5]   Chams-Davatchi, C., Valikhani, M., Daneshpazhooh, M., Esmaili, N., Balighi, K., Hallaji, Z., Barzegari, M., Akhiani, M., Ghodsi, Z., Mortazavi, H., Naraghi, Z. 2005. Pemphigus: Analysis of 1209 cases. *Int. J. Dermatol.* 44, 470-76.

[6]   Wilson, C.L., Wojnarowska, F., Dean, D., Pasricha, J.S.1993. IgG subclasses in pemphigus in Indian and UK populations. *Clin. Exp. Dermatol.* 18, 226-30.

[7]   Meyer, N., Misery, L. 2010. Geoepidemiologic considerations of auto-immune pemphigus. *Autoimm. Rev.* 9, A379-82.

[8]   Carson, P.J., Hameed, A., Ahmed, A.R. 1996. Influence of treatment on the clinical course of pemphigus vulgaris. *J. Am. Acad. Dermatol.* 34, 645-52.

[9]   V´lckova-Laskoska, M.T., Laskoski, D.S., Kamberova, S., Caca-Biljanovska, N., Volckova, N. 2007. Epidemiology of pemphigus in Macedonia: A 15-year retrospective study (1990-2004). *Int. J. Dermatol.* 46, 253-58.

[10]   Hahn-Ristic, K., Rzany,B., Amagai, M., Bröcker, E.B., Zillikens, D. 2002. Increased incidence of pemphigus vulgaris in southern European living in Germany compared with native Germans. *J. Eur. Acad. Dermatol. Venereol.*16, 68-71.

[11]   Gupta, V.K., Kelbel, T.E., Nguyen, D., Melonakos, K., Murrell, D.F., Xie, Y., Mullard, A., Reed, P.L., Seiffert-Sinha, K., Sinha, A. 2011. A globally available Internet-based patient survey of pemphigus vulgaris: Epidemiology and disease characteristics. *Dermatol. Clin.* 29, 393-404.

[12]   Bastuji-Garin, S., Souissi, R., Blum, L., Turki, H., Nouira, R., Jomaa, B., Zahaf, A., Ben Osman A., Mokhtar, I., Fazaa, B., Revuz, J., Roujeau, J.C, Kamoun, M.R. 1996.

Comparative epidemiology of pemphigus in Tunisia and France. Incidence of foliaceus pemphigus in young Tunisian women. *Ann. Dermatol. Venereol.* 123, 337-42.

[13] Micali, G., Musumeci, M.L., Nasca, M.R. 1998. Epidemiologic analysis and clinical course of 84 consecutive cases of pemphigus in eastern Sicily. *Int. J. Dermatol.* 37, 197-200.

[14] Tsankov, N., Vassilieva, S., Kamarashev, J., Kazandljeva, J., Kuzeva, V. 2000. Epidemiology of pemphigus in Sofia, Bulgaria. A 16-year retrospective study (1980-1995). *Int. J. Dermatol.* 39, 104-8.

[15] Svecova, D., Parnicka, Z., Pastyrikova, L., Urbancek, S., Luha, J., Buc, M. 2014. HLA DRB1* and DQB1* alleles are associated with disease severity in patients with pemphigus vulgaris. *Int. J. Dermatol.* doi: 10.1111/ijd. 12418.

[16] Uzun, S., Durdu, M., Akman, A., Akman, A., Gunasti, S., Uslular, C., Menisoglu, H.R., Alpsoy, E. 2006. Pemphigus in the Mediterranean region of Turkey: A study of 148 cases. *Int. J. Dermatol.* 45, 523-28.

[17] Seo, P.G., Choi, W.W., Chung, J.H. 2003. Pemphigus in Korea: clinical manifestations and treatment protocol. *J. Dermatol.* 30, 782-88.

[18] Zhu, X., Pan, J., Yu, Z., Wang, Y., Cai, L, Zheng, S. 2014. Epidemiology of pemphigus vulgaris in the Northeast China: a 10-year retrospective study. *J. Dermatol.* 41, 70-75.

[19] Mimouni,D., Bar, H., Gdalevich, M., Katzenelson, M.D. 2010. Pemphigus, analysis of 155 patients. *J. Eur. Acad. Dermatol. Venereol.* 24, 947-52.

[20] Mahajan,V.K., Sharma, N.L., Sharma, R.C., Garg, G. 2005. Twelve-year clinic-therapeutic experience in pemphigus: a retrospective study of 54 cases. *Int. J. Dermatol.* 44, 821-27.

[21] Marazza, G., Pham, H.C., Schärer, L., Pedrazzetti, P.P., Hunziker, T., Trüeb, R.M., Hohl, D., Itin, P., Lautenschlager, S., Naldi, L., Borradori, L. 2009. Incidence of bullous pemphigoid and pemphigus in Switzerland: a 2-year prospective study. *Br. J. Dermatol.*161, 861-68.

[22] Ljubojevic, S., Lipozencic, J., Brenner, S., Budimcic, D. 2002. Pemphigus vulgaris: a review of treatment over a 19-year period. *J. Eur. Acad. Dermatol. Venereol.* 16, 599-603.

[23] Alsaleh, Q.A., Nanda, A., Al-Baghli, N.M., Dvorak, R. 1999. Pemphigus in Kuwait. *Int. J. Dermatol.* 38, 351-56.

[24] Khaled, A., Ben Taazayet, S., Ben Alaya, N., Souissi, A., Zegloui, F., Kaffel, N., Kharfi, M., Zermani, R., Fazza, B. 2011. The course and prognosis of pemphigus in 47 Tunisian patients. *J. Eur. Acad. Dermatol. Venereol.* 27, 81-85.

[25] Ishii, N., Maeyama, Y., Karashima, T., Nakama, T., Kusuhara, M., Yasumoto, S., Hashimoto, T. 2008. A clinical study of patients with pemphigus vulgaris and pemphigus foliaceus: an 11-year retrospective study (1996-2006). *Clin. Exp. Dermatol.* 33, 641-43.

[26] Tallab, T, Joharji, H., Bahamdan, K., Karkashan, E., Mourad, M., Ibrahim, K. 2001. The incidence of pemphigus in the southern region of Saudi Arabia. *Int. J. Dermatol.* 40,570-72.

[27] Coronel-Peréz, I.M., Rodríguez-Rey, A.M., Pérez-Bernal, A.M., Camacho, F.M. 2009. Epidemiology of pemphigus in Hospital Universitario Virgen Macarena, Seville, Spain, 2005-2006. *Actas Dermosifiliogr.*100, 121-25.

[28] Alcaide-Martin, A.J., Gallardo-Pérez, M.A., Castillo-Munoz, R., Mendiola Fernández, M.V., Herrera-Ceballos, E. 2010. Epidemiologic study of 20 cases of pemphigus at Hospital Clinical Universitario Virgen de la Victoria de Málaga, Spain. 2010. *Actas Dermosifiliogr.* 101, 524-533.

[29] Rivera, R., Postigo, C., de la Mano, D., Vanaclocha, F., Iglesias, L. 2004. Penfigo: studio retrospective de 52 casos. *Actas Dermosifiliogr.* 95, 213-18.

[30] Woldegiorgis, S., Swerlick, R.A. 2001. Pemphigus in the Southeastern United States. *South. Med. J.* 94, 694:98.

[31] Naldi, L., Bertoni, M., Cainelli, T. 1993. Feasibility of a registry of pemphigus in Italy: two years experience. Gruppo Italiano Studi Epidemiologici in Dermatologia (GISED). *Int. J. Dermatol.* 6, 424-27.

[32] Michailidou, E.Z, Belazi, M.A., Markopoulos, A.K, Tsatsos, M.I., Mourellou, O.N., Antoniades, D.Z. 2007. Epidemiologic survey of pemphigus vulgaris with oral manifestations in northern Greece: retrospective study of 129 patients. *Int. J. Dermatol.* 46, 356-61.

[33] Svecova, D. 2014. Pemphigus vulgaris: a clinical study of 44 cases over a 20-year period. *Int. J. Dermatol.* doi10.1111/ijd.12644.

[34] Brenner, S., Wohl, Y. 2007. A survey of sex differences in 249 pemphigus patients and possible explanation. *Skinmed* 6, 163-65.

[35] Wandstrat, A., Wakeland, E. 2001. The genetics of complex autoimmune diseases: non-MHC susceptibility genes. *Nat. Immunol.* 2, 802-9.

[36] Humbert, P., Dupond, J.L., Vuitton, D., Agache, P. 1989. Dermatological autoimmune disease and the multiple autoimmune syndromes. *Acta Derm. Venereol. Suppl. (Stockh).* 148, 1-8.

[37] Leshem, Y.A., Katzenelson, V., Yosipovitch, G., David, M., Mimouni, D. 2011. Autoimmune disease in patients with pemphigus and their first-degree relatives. *Int. J. Dermatol.* 50, 827-31.

[38] Feinstein, A., Yorav, S., Movshovitz, M., Schewach-Millet, M. 1991. Pemphigus in families. *Int. J. Dermatol.* 30, 347-51.

[39] Ahmed, A.R., Sofen, H. 1982. Familial occurrence of pemphigus vulgaris. *Arch. Dermatol.* 118, 423-24.

[40] Starzycki, Z., Chorzelski, T.P., Jablonska, S. 1998. Familial pemphigus vulgaris in mother and daughter. *Int. J. Dermatol.* 37, 211-214.

[41] Bhol, K., Yunis, J., Ahmed, R.1996. Pemphigus vulgaris in distant relative of two families: association with major histocompatibility complex class II. *Clin. Exp. Dermatol.* 21, 100-103.

[42] Sinha, A.A. 2011. The genetics of pemphigus. *Dermatol. Clin.*29, 381-391.

[43] Firooz, A., Mazhar, A., Ahmed, A.R. 1994. Prevalence of autoimmune disease in the family members of patients with pemphigus vulgaris. *J. Am. Acad. Dermatol.* 31, 434-37.

[44] Doan, T., Melvold, R., Viselli, S., Waltenbaugh, C. 2013. Lippincott´s illustrated reviews: Immunology. Chapter 16 Autoimmunity. 2nd edition. Philadelphia, Wolters Kluwer/Lippincott Williams &Wilkins. 243-256.

[45] Scharf, S.J., Friedmann, A., Brautbar, C., Szafer, F., Steinman, L., Horn, G., Gyllenstein, U., Erlich, H.A. HLA class II allelic variation and susceptibility to pemphigus vulgaris. *Proc. Natl. Acad. Sci. USA.* 85, 3504-08.

[46] Todd, J.A., Acha-Orbea, H., Bell, J.I., Chao, N., Fronek, Z., Jacob, C.O., McDermott. M., Sinha, A.A, Timmeman, L., Steinman, L. 1988. A molecular basis for MHC class II-associated autoimmunity. *Science* 240, 1003-09.

[47] Niizeki, H., Inoko H., Mizuki N., Inamoto, N., Watababe, K., Hashimoto, T., Nishikawa, T. 1994. HLA-DQA1, -DQB1 and -DRB1 genotyping in Japanese pemphigus vulgaris patients by the PCR-RFLP method. *Tissue Antigens* 44, 248-51.

[48] Birol,A., Anadolu, R.Y., Tutkak, H., Gürgey, E. 2002. HLA-class 1 and class 2 antigens in Turkish patients with pemphigus. *Int. J. Dermatol.* 41, 79-83.

[49] Lee, E., Lendas, K.A., Chow, S., Pirani, Y., Gordon, D., Dionisio, R., Nquyen, D., Spizuoco, A., Fotino, M., Zhang, Y., Sinha, A.A. 2006. Disease relevant HLA class II alleles isolated by genotypic, haplotypic, and sequence analysis in North American Caucasians with pemphigus vulgaris. *Hum. Immunol.*67, 125-39.

[50] Loiseau, P., Lecleach, L., Prost, C., Lepage, V., Busson, M., Bustuji-Garin, S., Roujeau, J.C., Charron, D. 2000. HLA class polymorphism contributes to specify desmoglein derived peptides in pemphigus vulgaris and pemphigus foliaceus. *J. Autoimmun.* 15, 67-73.

[51] Lombardi, M.L., Mercuro, O., Tecame, G., Fusco, C., Ruocco, V., Salerno, A., Pirozzi, G., Manzo, C. 1996. Molecular analysis of HLA DRB1 and DQB1 in Italian patients with pemphigus vulgaris. *Tissue antigens* 47, 228-30.

[52] Gonzáles-Escribano, M.F., Jiménez, G., Walter, K., Perez-Bernal, A.M., Rodriguez, M.R., Conejo-Mir, J.S., Núnez-Roldán, A.1998. Distribution of HLA class II alleles among Spanish patients with pemphigus vulgaris. *Tissue Antigens* 52, 275-78.

[53] Glorio, R., Rodriguez Costa, G., Haas, R., Gruber, M., Faiboim, L., Woscoff, A. 2002. HLA haplotypes and class II molecular alleles in Argentinian patients with pemphigus vulgaris. *J. Cutan. Med. Surg.* 6, 422-26.

[54] Mobini, N., Yunis, E.J., Alper, C.A., Yunis, J.J., Delgado, J.C., Yunis, D.E., Firooz. A., Dowlati, Y., Bahar, K., Gregersen, P.K., Ahmed, A.R. 1997. Identical MHC markers in non-Jewish Iranian and Ashkenazi Jewish patients with pemphigus vulgaris: a possible common central Asian ancestral origin. *Hum. Immunol.* 15, 62-67.

[55] Miygawa, S., Niizeki, H., Yamashina, Y., Kaneshige, T. 2002. Genotyping for HLA A, B and C alleles in Japanese patients with pemphigus: prevalence of Asian alleles of the HLA-B15 family. *Br. J. Dermatol.* 146, 52-58.

[56] Harfouch, E., Daoud, S. 2014. Allelic variation in HLA-DRB1* loci in Syrian pemphigus vulgaris patients. *Int. J. Dermatol.* Doi 10.1111/ijd.12184.

[57] Delgado, J.C., Hameed, A., Yunis, J.J., Bhol, K., Rojas, A.L., Rehman, S.B., Khan, A.A., Ahmad, M., Alper, C.A., Ahmed, A.R., Yunis, E.J. 1997. Pemphigus vulgaris autoantibody response is linked to HLA-DQB1*0503 in Pakistani patients. *Hum. Immunol.* 57, 110-19.

[58] Zhou, S.H., Lin, L., Jin, P.Y., Ye, S.Z. 2003. Association between HLA-DRB1, DQB1 gens and pemphigus vulgaris in Chinese Hans. *Zhonghua Yi Xue Yi Chuan Xue Za Zhi.* 20, 79-81.

[59] Koc, C.K., Sallakci, N., Akman-Karakas, A., Alpsoy, E., Yegin, O. 2013. Human leukocyte antigens class I and class II in patients with pemphigus in southern Turkey. *Int. J. Dermatol.* 52, 53-58.

[60] Tunca, M., Musabak, U., Sagkan, I., Koc, E., Akar, A. 2010. Association of human leukocyte antigen class II alleles with pemphigus vulgaris in a Turkish population. *J. Dermatol.* 37, 246-50.

[61] Delgado, J.C., Yunis, D.E., Bozón, M.V., Salazar, M., Deulofeut, R., Turbay, D., Mehra, N.K., Pasricha, J.S., Raval, R.S., Patel, H., Shah, B.K., Bhol, K., Alper, C.A., Ahmed, A.R., Yunis, E.J. 1996. MHC class II alleles and haplotypes in patients with pemphigus vulgaris from India. *Tissue Antigens* 48, 668-72.

[62] Marsh, S.G., Albert, E.D., Bodmer, W.F., Bontrop, R.E., Dupont, B., Erlich, H,A, Fernández-Vina, M., Geraghty, D.E., Holdsworth, R., Hurley, C.K., Lau, M., Lee, K.W., Mach, B., Maiers, M., Mayr, W.R., Müller, C.R., Parham, P., Petersdorf, E.W., Sasazuki, T., Strominger, J.L., Svejgaard, A., Terasaki, P.I., Tiercy, J.M., Trowsdale, J. 2010. Nomenclature for the HLA system 2010. *Tissue Antigens* 75, 291-455.

[63] Slomov, E., Loewenthal, R., Goldberg, I., Korostihenvsky, M., Brenner, S., Gazit, E. 2003. Pemphigus vulgaris in Jewish patients is associated with HLA-A region genes: mapping by microsatellite markers. *Hum. Immunol.* 64, 771-79.

[64] Lombardi, M.L., Mercuro, O., Ruocco, V., Lo Schiavo, A., Lombari,V., Guerrera, V., Pirozzi, G., Manzo, C. 1999. Common human leukocyte antigen alleles in pemphigus vulgaris and pemphigus foliaceus Italian patients. *J. Invest. Dermatol.* 113, 107-10.

[65] Carcassi, C., Cottoni, F., Floris, L., Vacca, A., Mulargia, M., Arras, M., Boero, R., La Nasa, G., Ledda, A., Pizzati, A., Cerimele, D., Contu, L.1996. HLA haplotypes and class II molecular alleles in Sardinian and Italian patients with pemphigus vulgaris. *Tissue Antigens* 48, 662-67.

[66] Glorio, R.R., Rodriguez Costa, G., Haas, R., Larriba, J., Fainboim, L., Woscoff, A. 1999. PCR determination of an association between class II HLA and pemphigus vulgaris. *Medicina (B Aires)* 59, 28-32.

[67] Shams, S., Amirzargar, A.A., Yousefi, M., Rezaei, N., Solgi, G., Khosravi, F., Ansaripour, B., Moradi, B., Nikbin, B. 2009. HLA class II (DRB, DQA1 and DQB1) allele and haplotype frequencies in the patients with pemphigus vulgaris. *J. Clin. Immunol.* 29, 175-79.

[68] Miyagawa, S., Higashimine, I., Lida, T., Yamashina, Y., Fukumoto, T., Shirai, T. 1997. HLA-DRB1*4 and DRB*14 alleles are associated with susceptibility to pemphigus among Japanese. *J. Invest. Dermatol.* 109, 615-18.

[69] Weber, R., Monteiro, F., Preuhs-Filho, G., Rodrigues, H., Kalil, J., Miziara, D. 2011. HLA-DRB1*04:02, DRB1*08:04 and DRB1*14 alleles associated to pemphigus vulgaris in Southeastern Brazilian population. *Tissue Antigen* 78, 92-93.

[70] Albis-Camps, M., Bunce, M., Blasczyk, R., Horn, P.A. 2006. DRB*1454 is the most frequent DRB*14 allele. *Hum. Immunol.* 67 (Suppl1), S114.

[71] Marsh, S.G., WHO Nomenclature Committee for Factors of the HLA System.2006. Nomenclature for factors of the HLA system, update October 2005. *Tissue Antigens* 67, 258-59.

[72] Yang, K.L., Chen, M.J., Lee, S.K., Lin, C.C., Tsai, M.J., Chiu, H.M., Jiang, S., Chao, Y.C., Chen, S.P., Lin, S., Shyr, M.H, Lin, P.Y. 2009. New allele name of some HLA-DRB1*1401: HLA-DRB1*1454. *Int. J. Immunogenet.* 36, 119-20.

[73] Horn, P,A., Albis-Camps, M., Verboom, M., Bunce, M., Yousaf, K., Williams, S., Blasczyk. 2007. The nature of diversity of HLA-DRB1 exon 3. *Tissue Antigens* 70, 335-37.

[74] Saha, M., Harman, K., Mortimer, N.J., Binda, V., Black, M.M., Kondeatis, E., Vaughan, R., Groves, R.W. 2010. Pemphigus vulgaris in white Europeans is linked with HLA class II allele HLA DRB1*1454 but not DRB1*1401. *J. Invest. Dermatol.* 130, 311-14.

[75] Párnická, Z., Švecová, D., Javor, J., Shawkatová, I., Buc, M. 2013. High susceptibility to pemphigus vulgaris due to HLA-DRB1*14:54 in the Slovak population. *Int. J. Immunogenet.* 40, 471-78.

[76] Buc, M., Párnická, Z., Švecová, D., Pastyriková, L. 2012. Different association of HLA-DR and DQ alleles in Slovak Caucasoid and Romany pemphigus vulgaris patients: a preliminary report. 8th International Congress on Autoimmunity, Granada Spain, Abstract book (CD) 211.

[77] Ruiz-Morales, J.A., Vargas-Alarcón, G., Flores-Villanueva, P.O., Villarreal-Garza, C., Hernández-Pacheco, G., Yamamoto-Furusho, J.K., Rodríguez-Pérez, J.M., Pérez-Hernández, H., Rull, M., Cardiel, M.H., Granados, J. 2004. HLA-DRB1 alleles encoding the "shared epitope" are associated with susceptibility to developing rheumatoid arthritis whereas HLA-DRB1 alleles encoding an aspartic acid at position 70 of beta-chain are protective in Mexican Mestizos. *Hum. Immunol.* 65, 262-69.

[78] Al-Hussein, K.A., Rama, N.R., Ahmad, M., Rozemuller, E., Tilanus, M.G. 2003. HLA-DPB1*0401 is associated with dominant protection against type 1 diabetes in the general Saudi population and subjects with a high-risk DR/DQ haplotype. *Eur. J. Immunogenet.* 30, 115-19.

[79] The International Multiple Sclerosis Genetics Consortium (IMSGC), Wellcome Trust case Control Consortium. 2012. Genetic risk and a primary role for cell-mediated immune mechanisms in multiple sclerosis. *Nature* 476 (7359), 214-19.

[80] Marchini, M., Antonioli, R., Lleó, A., Barili, M., Caronnin, M., Origgi, L., Vanoli, M., Scorza, R. 2003. HLA class II antigens associated with lupus nephritis in Italian SLE patients. *Hum. Immunol.* 64, 462-68.

[81] Chen, Q.Y., Huang, W., She, J.X., Baxter, F., Volpe, R., Maclaren, N.K. 1999. HLA-DRB1*08, DRB1*03/DRB3*0101, and DRB3*0202 are susceptibility genes for Graves´ disease in North American Caucasians, whereas DRB1*07 is protective. *J. Clin. Endocrinol. Metab.* 84, 3182-86.

[82] Yan, L., Wang, J.M., Zeng, K. 2012. Association between HLA-DRB1 polymorphisms and pemphigus vulgaris: a meta-analysis. *Br. J. Dermatol.* 167, 768-77.

[83] Sanjeevi, C.B. 2000. HLA-DQ6-mediated protection in IDDM. *Hum. Immunol.* 61, 148-53.

[84] Geng, L., Wang, Y., Zhai, N., Lu, Y.N., Song, F.J., Chen, H.D. 2005. Association between pemphigus vulgaris and human leukocyte antigen in Han nation of northeast China. *Clin. Med. Sci.* J. 20, 166-70.

[85] Hashimoto, K., Miki, Y., Nakata, S., Matsuyama, M. 1977. HLA-10 in pemphigus among Japanese. *Arch. Dermatol.*113, 1518-19.

[86] Ahmed, A.R., Yunis, E.J., Khatri, K., Wagner, R., Notani, G., Awdeh, Z., Alper, C.A. 1990. Major histocompatibility complex haplotypes studies in Ashkenazi Jewish patients with pemphigus vulgaris. *Proc. Natl. Acad. Sci. U. S. A.* 87, 7658-62.

[87] Bhanusali, D.G., Sachev, A., Rahmanian, A., Gerlach, J.A., Tong, J.C., Seifert-Sinha, K., Sinha, A.A. 2013. HLA-E*0103X is associated with susceptibility to pemphigus vulgaris. *Exp. Dermatology* 22, 108-12.

[88]   Park, K. S., Park, J. S., Nam, J. H., Bang, D., Sohn, S., Lee, E.S. 2007. HLA-E*0101
       and HLA-G*010101reduce the risk of Behcet´s disease. *Tisue Antigens* 69, 139-44.

[89]   Gazit, E., Somov, Y., Goldberg, I., Brenner, S., Loewenthal, R. 2004. HLA-G is
       associated with pemphigus vulgaris in Jewish patients. *Hum. Immunol.* 65, 39-46.

[90]   Ishitani, A., Geraghty, D.E. 1992. Alternative splicing of HLA-G transcripts yields
       proteins with primary structures resembling both class I and class II antigens. *Proc.
       Natl. Acad. U.S.A.* 89, 3947-51.

[91]   Le Bouteiller, P., Solier, C. 2001. Is antigen presentation the primary function of HLA-
       G? *Microbes Infect.* 3, 323-32.

[92]   Capon, F., Trembath, R.C., Harman, K.E. 2006. Evidence of an association between
       desmoglein 3 haplotypes and pemphigus vulgaris. *Br. J. Dermatol.* 154, 67-71.

[93]   Gibson, W.T., Walter, M.A., Ahmed, A.R., Alper, C.A., Cox, D.W. 1994. The
       immunoglobulin heavy chain and disease association: application to pemphigus
       vulgaris. *Hum. Genet.* 94, 675-83.

[94]   Zitouni, M., Martel, P., Ben Ayed, M., Raux, G., Gilbert, D., Joly, P., Mokhtar, I.,
       Kamoun, M.R., Turki, H., Zahaf, A., Mokni, M., Ben Osman, A., Masmoudi, H.,
       Makni, S., Tron, F. 2002. Pemphigus is not associated with allotypic markers of
       immunoglobulin kappa. *Genes Immun.* 3, 50-52.

[95]   Nizeki, H., Kumagai, S., Kanagawa, S., Amagai, M., Yamashina, Y., Asada, H.,
       Nishikawa, S. 2004. Exclusion of the TAP1 and TAP2 genes within the HLA class II
       region as candidate susceptibility genes to pemphigus in the Japanese population. *J.
       Dermatol. Sci.* 36, 122-24.

[96]   Bidwell, J., Keen, L., Gallagher, G., Kimberly, R., Huizinga, T., McDermott, M.F.,
       Oksenberg, J., McNicholl, J., Pociot, F., Hardt, C., D´Alfonso, S. 1999. Cytokine gene
       polymorphism in human disease: on-line databases. *Genes Immun.* 1, 3-19.

[97]   Hollegaard, M.V., Bidwell, J.L. 2006. Cytokine gene polymorphism in human disease:
       on-line databases. *Genes Immun.* 7, 269-76.

[98]   Javor, J., Chmurova, N., Parnicka, Z., Ferencik, S., Grosse-Wilde, H, Buc, M.,
       Svecova, D. 2010. TNF-α and IL-10 gene polynorphisms show a weak association
       with pemphigus vulgaris in the Slovak population. *J. Eur. Acad. Dermatol. Venereol.*
       24, 65-68.

[99]   Eberhard, Y., Burgos, E., Gagliardi, J., Vullo, C.M., Borosky, A., Pesoa, S., Serra,
       H.M. 2005. Cytokine polymorphisms in patients with pemphigus. *Arch. Dermatol. Res.*
       296, 309-13.

[100] Bhol, K.C., Rojas, A.I., Khan, I.U., Ahmed, A.R. 2000. Presence of interleukin 10 in
       the serum and blister fluid of patients with pemphigus vulgaris and pemphigoid.
       Cytokine 12, 1076-83.

[101] Toto, P., Feliciani, C., Amerio, P., Suzuki, H., Wang, B., Shivji, G.M., Woodley, D.,
       Sauder, D. 2000. Immune modulation in pemphigus vulgaris: role of CD28 and IL-10.
       J. Immunol. 164, 522-29.

[102] D´Auria, L., Bonifaci, C., Mussi, A., D´Agosto, G., De Simone, C., Giacalone, B.,
       Ferraro, C., Ameglio, F. 1997. Cytokines in the sera of patients with pemphigus
       vulgaris: interleukin-6 and tumor necrosis factor-alpha levels are significantly
       increased as compared to healthy subjects and correlate with disease activity. *Eur.
       Cytokine Netw.* 8, 383-87.

[103] Feliciani, C., Toto, P., Amerio, P., Pour, S.M., Coscione, G., Amerio, P., Shivji, G., Wang, B., Sauder, D.N. 1999. *In vitro* and *In vivo* Expression of interleukin-1α and tumor necrosis factor -α are involved in acantholysis. 2000. *J. Invest. Dermatol.* 114, 71-77.

[104] Lopéz-Robles, E., Avalos-Díaz, E., Vega-Memije, E., Hojyo-Tomoka, T., Villalobos, R., Fraire, S., Domíguez-Soto, L., Herrera-Esparza, R. 2001. TNFα and IL-6 are mediators in the blistering process of pemphigus. *Int. J. Dermatol.* 40, 185-88.

[105] Feliciani, C., Toto, P., Wang, B., Sauder, D.N., Amerio, P., Tulli, A. 2003. Urokinase plasminogen activator mRNA is induced by IL-1α and TNF-α in *in vitro* acantholysis. *Exp. Dermatol.* 12, 466-71.

[106] Torzecka, J.D., Narbutt, J., Sysa-Jedrzejowska, A., Borowiec, M., Ptasinska, A., Woszczek, G., Kowalski, M. 2003. Tumor necrosis factor-α polymorphism as one of the complex inherited factors in pemphigus. *Mediators Inflamm.*12, 303-7.

[107] Michou, L., Lasbleiz, S., Rat, A.C., Migliorini, P., Balsa, A., Westhovens, R., Barrera, P., Alves, H., Pierlot, C., Glikmans, E., Garnier, S., Dausset, J., Vaz, C., Fernandes, M., Petit-Teixeira, E., Lemaire, I., Pascual-Salcedo, D., Bombardieri, S., Dequeker, J., Radstake, T.R., Van Riel, P., van de Putte, L., Lopes-Vaz, A., Prum, B., Bardin, T., Dieudé, P., Cornélis, F. 2007. Linkage proof for PTPN22, a rheumatoid arthritis susceptibility gene and human autoimmunity gene. *Proc. Natl. Acad. Sci.U.S.A.*104, 1649-54.

[108] Howson, J.M., Dunger, D.B., Nutland, S.A., Stevens, H., Wicker, L.S., Todd, J.A. 2007. A type 1 diabetes subgroup with a female bias is characterised by failure in tolerance to thyroid peroxidase at an early age and a strong association with the cytotoxic T-lymphocyte-associated antigen-4 gene. *Diabetologia* 50, 741-46.

[109] Balada, E., Villarreal-Tolchinsky, J., Ordi-Ros, J., Labrador, M., Serrano-Acedo, S., Martinez-Lostao,L., Vilardell-Tarrés, M. 2006. Multiplex family-based study in systemic lupus erythematosus: association between the R620W polymorphism of PTPN22 and the FcgammaRIIa (CD32A) R131 allele. *Tissue Antigens* 68, 432-38.

[110] Sachdev, A., Bhanusali, D.G., Patterson, K.C., Zamora, M.B., Ghuman, A., Gerlach, J.A., Sinha, A.A. 2011. PTPN22 1858T is not a risk factor for North American pemphigus vulgaris. *Exp. Dermatol.* 20, 514-19.

[111] Dhandha, M.M., Seiffert-Sinha, K., Sinha, A.A. 2012. Specific immunoglobulin isotypes correlate with disease activity, morphology, duration and HLA association in pemphigus vulgaris. *Autoimmunity* 45, 516-26.

[112] Waschke, J. 2008. The desmosome and pemphigus. *Histochem. Cell. Biol.* 130, 21-54.

[113] Skerrow, C.J., Clelland, D.G., Skerrow, D. 1989. Changes to desmosomal antigens and lectin-binding sites during differentiation in normal human epidermis: a quantitative ultrastructural study. *J. Cell. Sci.* 92, 667-77.

[114] North, A.J., Bardsley, W.G., Hyam, J., Bornslaeger, E.A., Cordingley, H.C., Trinnaman, B., Hatzfeld, M., Green, K.J., Magee, A.I., Garrod, D.R.1999. Molecular map of the desmosomal plaque. *J. Cell. Sci.* 112, 4325-36.

[115] Kitajima, Y. 2013. New insight into desmosome regulation and pemphigus blistering as a desmosome-remodeling disease. *Kaohsiung J. Med. Sci.* 29, 1-13.

[116] Buxton, R.S., Cowin, P., Franke, W.W., Garrod, D.R., Green, K.J., King, I.A., Koch, P.J., Magee, A.I., Rees, D.A., Stanley, J.R., Steinberg, M.S. 1993. Nomenclature of the Desmosomal Cadherins. *J. Cell. Biol.* 121, 481-83.

[117] Kjuic, A., Bazzi, H., Sundberg, J.P., Martinez-Mir, A., O´Shaughnessy, R., Mahoney, M.G., Levy, M., Montagutelli, X., Ahmad, W., Aita, V.M., Gordon, D., Uitto, J., Whiting, D., Ott, J., Fisher, S., Gilliam, T.C., Jahoda, C.A., Morris, R.J., Panteleyev, A.A., Nguyen, V.T., Christiano, A.M. 2003. Desmoglein 4 in hair follicle differentiation and epidermal adhesion: evidence from inherited hypotrichosis and acquired pemphigus vulgaris. *Cell* 133, 249-60.

[118] Pilichou, K., Nava, A., Basso, C., Beffagna, G., Bauce, B., Lorenzon, A., Frigo, G., Vettori, A., Valente, M., Towbin, J., Thiene, G., Danieli, G.A., Rampazzo, A. 2006. Mutation in desmoglein-2 gene is associated with arrhythmogenic right ventricular cardiomyopathy. *Circulation* 113, 1171-79.

[119] Koch, P.J., Mahoney, M.G., Ishikawa, H., Pulkkinen, L., Uitto, J., Shultz, L., Murphy, G.F., Whitaker-Menezes, D., Stanley, J.R. 1997. Targeted disruption of the pemphigus vulgaris antigen (desmoglein 3) gene in mice causes loss of keratinocyte cell adhesion with a phenotype similar to pemphigus vulgaris. *J. Cell. Biol.* 137, 1091-102.

[120] Dusek, R.L., Godsel, L.M., Green, K.J. 2007. Discriminating roles of desmosomal cadherins: beyond desmosomal adhesion. *J. Dermatol. Sci.* 45, 7-21.

[121] Garrod, D., Chidgey, M. 2008. Desmosome structure, composition and function. *Biochim. Biophys. Acta* 1178, 578-87.

[122] Spinder, V., Heupel, W.M., Efthymiadis, A., Schmidt, E., Eming, R., Rank, C., Hinterdorfer, P., Müller, T., Drenckhahn, D., Waschke, J. 2009. Desmocollin 3-mediated binding is crucial for keratinocyte cohesion and is impaired in pemphigus. *J. Biol. Chem.* 284, 30556-64.

[123] Cownin, P., Kapprell, H.P., Franke, W.W., Tamkun, J., Hynes, R.O. 1986. Plakoglobin: a protein common to different kinds of intercellular adhering junctions. *Cell* 46, 1063-73.

[124] Chitaev, N.A., Averbakh, A.Z., Troyanovsky, R.B., Troyanovsky, S.M. 1998. Molecular organization of the desmoglein-plakoglobin complex. *J. Cell. Sci.* 30, 1941-49.

[125] Bonné, S., Gilbert, B., Hatzfeld, M., Chen, X., Green, K.J., van Roy, F. 2003. Defining desmosomal plakophilin-3 interactions. *J. Cell. Biol.* 161, 403-16.

[126] Bierkamp, C., Mclaughlin, K.J., Schwarz, H., Huber, O., Kemler, R. 1996. Embryonic heart and skin defects in mice lacking plakoglobin. *Dev. Biol.* 180, 780-85.

[127] Maeda, O., Usami, N., Kondo, M., Takahashi, M., Goto, H., Shimokata, K., Kusugami, K., Sekido, Y. 2004. Plakoglobin (gamma-catenin) has TCF/LEF family-dependent transcriptional activity in beta-catenin-deficient cell line. *Oncogene* 23, 964-72.

[128] Williamson, L., Raess, N.A., Caldelari, R., Zakher, A., de Bruin, A., Posthaus, H., Bolli, R, Hunziker, T., Suter, M.M., Müller, E.J. 2006. Pemphigus vulgaris identifies plakoglobin as key suppressor of c-Myc in the skin. *EMBO J.* 25, 3298-309.

[129] Dusek, R.L., Godsel, L.M., Chen, F., Strohecker, A.M., Getsios, S., Harmon, R., Müller, E.J., Caldelari, R., Cryns, V.L., Green, K.J. 2007. Plakoglobin deficiency protects keratinocytes from apoptosis. *J. Invest. Dermatol.* 127, 792-801.

[130] Kowalczyk, A.P., Bornslaeger, E.A., Norvell, S.M., Palka, H.L., Green, K.J. 1999. Desmosomes: intercellular adhesive junctions specialized for attachment of intermediate filaments. *Int. Rev. Cytol.* 185, 237-302.

[131] Chitaev, N.A., Leube, R.E., Troayanovsky, R.B., Eshkind, L.G., Franke, W.W., Troyanovsky, S.M. 1996. The binding of plakoglobin to desmosomal cadherins: patterns of binding sites and topogenic potential. *J. Cell. Biol.* 133, 359-69.

[132] Wahl, J.K. 2005. A role for plakophilin-1 in the initiation of desmosome assembly. *J. Cell. Biochem.* 96, 390-403.

[133] Grossmann, K.S., Grund, C., Huelsken, J., Behrend, M., Erdmann, B., Franke, W.W., Birchmeier, W. 2004. Requirement of plakophilin 2 for heart morphogenesis and cardiac junction formation. *J. Cell. Biol.* 167, 149-160.

[134] Cirillo, N., AlShwaimi, E., McCullough, M., Prime, S.S. 2014. Pemphigus vulgaris autoimmune globulin induces Src-dependent tyrosine-phosphorylation of plakophilin 3 and its detachment from desmoglein 3. *Autoimmunity* 47, 134-40.

[135] Hatzfeld, M., Wolf, A., Keil, R. 2014. Plakophilins in desmosomal adhesion and signaling. *Cell. Commun. Adhes.* 21, 25-42.

[136] Smith, E.A., Fuchs, E. 1998. Defining the interactions between intermediate filaments and desmosomes. *J. Cell. Biol.* 141, 1229-41.

[137] Gallicano, G.I., Kouklis, P., Bauer, C., Yin, M., Vasioukhin, V., Degenstein, L., Fuchs, E. 1998. Desmoplakin is required early in development for assembly of desmosomes and cytoskeletal linkage. *J. Cell. Biol.* 143, 2009-22.

[138] Gallicano, I.G., Bauer, C., Fuchs, E. 2001. Rescuing desmoplakin function in extra-embryonic ectoderm reveals the importance of this protein in embryonic heart, neuroepithelium, skin and vasculature. *Development* 128, 929-41.

[139] Mahoney, M.G., Hu, Y., Brennan, D., Bazzi, H., Christiano, A.M., Wahl, J.K. 2006. Delineation of diversified desmoglein distribution in stratified squamous epithelia: implications in diseases. *Exp. Dermatol.* 15, 101-109.

[140] Kimura, T.E., Merritt, A.J., Garrod, D.R. 2007. Calcium-independent desmosomes of keratinocytes are hyperadhesive. *J. Invest. Dermatol.* 127, 775-81.

[141] Mattey, D.L., Garrod, D.R. 1986. Calcium-induced desmosome formation in cultured kidney epithelial cells. *J. Cell. Sci.* 85, 95-111.

[142] Garrod, D., Kimura, T.E. 2008. Hyper-adhesion: a new concept in cell-cell adhesion. *Biochem. Soc. Trans.* 36, 195-201.

[143] Garrod, D.R., Berika, M.Y., Bardsley, W.F., Holmes, D., Tabernero, L. 2005. Hyper-adhesion in desmosomes: its regulation in wound healing and possible relationship to cadherin crystal structure. *J. Cell. Sci.* 118, 5743-54.

[144] Yin, T., Getsios, S., Caldelari, R., Godsel, L.M., Kowalczyk, A., Müller, E.J., Green, K.J. 2005. Mechanism of plakoglobin-dependent adhesion. Desmosome specific functions in assembly and regulation by epidermal growth factor receptor. *J. Biol. Chem.* 280, 40355-63.

[145] Pokutta, S., Weis, W.I. 2007. Structure and mechanism of cadherines and catenins in cell-cell contacts. *Annu. Rev. Cell. Dev. Biol.* 23, 237-61.

[146] Mahoney, M.G., Wang, Z., Rothenberg, K., Koch, P.J., Amagai, M., Stanley, J.R. 1999. Explanations for the clinical and microscopic localization of lesions in pemphigus foliaceus and vulgaris. *J. Clin. Invest.* 103, 461-468.

[147] Amagai, M., Tsunoda, K., Zillikens, D., Nagai, T., Nishikawa, T. 1999. The clinical phenotype of pemphigus is defined by the anti-desmoglein autoantibody profile. *J. Am. Acad. Dermatol.* 40 (2 Pt 1), 167-70.

[148] Bystryn, J.C., Rudolph, J.L. 2005. Pemphigus. *Lancet* 366, 61-73.

[149] Spindler, V., Drenckhahn, D., Zillikens, D., Waschke, J. 2007. Pemphigus IgG causes skin splitting in the presence of both desmoglein 1 and desmoglein 3. *Am. J. Pathol.* 171, 906-16.

[150] Grando, S.A. 2012. Pemphigus autoimmunity: Hypothesis and realities. *Autoimmunity.* 45, 7-35.

[151] Ohyama, B., Nishifuji, K., Chan, P.T., Kawaguchi, A., Yamashita, T., Ishii, N., Hamada, T., Dainichi, T., Koga, H., Tsuruta, D., Amagaii, M., Hashimoto,T. 2012. Epitope spreading is rarely found in pemphigus vulgaris by large-scale longitudinal study using desmoglein 2-based swapped molecules. *J. Invest. Dermatol.* 132, 1158-68.

[152] Tchernev, G., Orfanos, C.E. 2006. Antigen mimicry, epitope spreading and the pathogenesis of pemphigus. *Tissue Antigens* 68, 280-86.

[153] Ishii, K., Amagai, M., Ohata, Y., Shimizu, H., Hashimoto, T., Ohya, K., Nishikawa, T. 2000. Development of pemphigus vulgaris in patients with pemphigus foliaceus: Antidesmoglein antibody profile shift confirmed by enzyme-linked immunosorbent assay. *J. Am. Acad. Dermatol.* 42, 859-61.

[154] Komai, A., Amagai, M., Ishii, K., Nishikawa, T., Chorzelski, T., Matsuo, I., Hashimoto, T. 2001. The clinical transition between pemphigus foliaceus and pemphigus vulgaris correlates well with the changes in autoantibody profile assessed by an enzyme-linked immunosorbent assay. *Br. J. Dermatol.* 144, 1177-82.

[155] Salato, V.K., Hacker-Foegen, M.K., Lazarova, Z., Fairley, J.A, Lin, M.S. 2005. Role of intramolecular epitope spreading in pemphigus vulgaris. *Clin. Immunol.* 116, 54-64.

[156] Li, N., Aoki, V., Hans-Filho, G., Rivitti, E.A., Diaz, L.A. 2003. The role of intramolecular epitope spreading in the pathogenesis of endemic pemphigus foliaceus (Fogo Selvagem). *J. Exp. Med.* 197, 1501-10.

[157] Chan, P.T., Ohyama, B., Nishifuji, K., Yoshida, K., Ishii, K., Hashimoto, T., Amagai, M. 2010. Immune response towards the amino-terminus of desmoglein 1 prevails across different activity stages in nonendemic pemphigus foliaceus. *Br. J. Dermatol.* 162, 1242-50.

[158] Joly, P., Litrowski, N. 2011. Pemphigus group (vulgaris, vegetans, foliaceus, herpetiformis, brasiliensis). *Clin. Dermatol.* 29, 432-23.

[159] Chen, J., Den, Z., Koch, P.J. 2008. Loss of desmocollin 3 in mice leads to epidermal blistering. *J. Cell. Sci.* 121, 2844-49.

[160] Nguyen, V.T., Chernyavsky, A.I., Arrendo, J., Bercovich, D., Orr-Urtreger, A., Vetter, D.E., Wess, J., Beaudet, A.L., Kitajima, Y., Grando, S.A. 2004. Synergistic control of keratinocyte adhesion through muscarinic and nicotinic acethylcholine receptor subtypes. *Exp. Cell. Res.* 294, 534-49.

[161] Nguyen, T.V., Ndoye, A., Grando, S.A. 2000. Novel human α9 acetylcholine receptor regulating keratinocyte adhesion is targeted by pemphigus vulgaris autoimmunity. *Am. J. Pathol.* 157, 1377-91.

[162] Nguyen, T.V., Ndoye, A., Grando, S.A. 2000. Pemphigus vulgaris antibody identifies pemphaxin. *J. Biol. Chem.* 275, 29466-76.

[163] Marchenko, S., Chernyavsky, A.I., Arredondo, J., Gindi, V., Grando, S.A. 2010. Antimitochondrial autoantibodies in pemphigus vulgaris. *J. Biol. Chem.* 285, 3695-704.

[164] Harman, K.E., Seed, P.T., Gratian, M.J., Bhogal, B.S., Challacombe, S.J., Black, M.M. 2001. The severity of cutaneous and oral pemphigus is related to desmoglein 1 and 3 antibody levels. *Br. J. Dermatol.* 144, 775-780.

[165] Herrero-González, J.E., Iranzo, P., Benitez, D., Lozano, F., Herrero, C., Mascaro, J.M. Jr. 2010. Correlation of immunological profile with phenotype and disease outcome in pemphigus. *Acta Derm. Venereol.* 90, 401-5.

[166] Malehi, A.S., Hajizadeh, E., Ahmadi, K., Mansouri, P., 2014. Assessing the autobody levels in relation to recurrence of pemphigus: joint modeling of longitudinal measurements and recurrent event times. *Iran. Red. Crescent Med. J.* 16, e13812.

[167] Schmidt, E., Dähnrich, C., Rosemann, A., Probst, C., Komorowski, L., Saschenbrecker, S., Schlumberger, W., Stöcker, W., Hashimoto, T., Bröcker, E.B., Recke, A., Rose, C., Zillikens, D. 2010. Novel ELISA systems for antibodies to desmoglein 1 and 3: correlation of disease activity with serum antibody levels in individual pemphigus patients. *Exp. Dermatol.* 19, 458-63.

[168] Avgerinou, G., Papafragkaki, D.K., Nasiopoulou, A., Markantoni, V., Arapaki, A., Servitzoglou, M., Katsambas, A., Stavropoulos, P.G. 2013. Correlation of antibodies against desmogleins 1 and 3 with indirect immunofluorescence and disease status in a Greek population with pemphigus vulgaris. *J. Eur. Acad. Dermatol. Venereol.* 27, 430-5.

[169] Wasserstrum, N., Laros, R.K. Jr. 1983. Transplacental transmission of pemphigus. *JAMA* 249, 1480-82.

[170] Anhalt, G.J., Labib, R.S., Voorhees, J.J., Beals, T.F., Diaz, L.A. 1982. Induction of pemphigus in neonatal mice by passive transfer of IgG from patients with the disease. *N. Engl. J. Med.* 306, 1189-96.

[171] Chowdhury, M.M., Natarajan, S. 1998. Neonatal pemphigus vulgaris associated with mild oral pemphigus vulgaris in the mother during pregnancy. *Br. J. Dermatol.* 139, 500-3.

[172] Rocha-Alvarez, R., Friedman, H., Campbell, I.T., Souza-Aguiar, L., Martins-Castro, R., Diaz, L.A. 1992. Pregnant women with endemic pemphigus foliaceus (Fogo Selvagem) give birth to disease-free babies. *J. Invest. Dermatol.* 99, 78-82.

[173] Abasq, C., Mouquet, H., Gilbert, D., Tron, F., Grassi, V., Musette, P., Joly, P.2009. ELISA testing of anti-desmoglein 1 and 3 antibodies in the management of pemphigus. *Arch. Dermatol.* 145, 529-35.

[174] Akman, A., Uzun, S., Alpsoy, E. 2010. Immunopathologic features of pemphigus in the east Mediterranean region of Turkey: a prospective study. *Skinmed* 8, 12-16.

[175] Belloni-Fortina, A., Faggion, D., Pigozzi, B., Peserico, A., Bordignon, M., Baldo, V., Alaibac, M. 2009. Detection of autoantibodies against recombinant desmoglein 1 and 3 molecules in patients with pemphigus vulgaris: correlation with disease extent at the time of diagnosis and during follow-up. *Clin. Dev. Immunol.* 2009, 187864.

[176] Khandpur, S., Sharma, V.K., Sharma, A., Pathria, G., Satyam, A. 2010. Comparison of enzyme-linked immunosorbent assay test with immunoblot assay in the diagnosis of Indian patients. *Indian. J. Dermatol. Venereol. Leprol.* 76, 27-32.

[177] Hilario-Vargas, J., Dasher, D., Li, N., Aoki, V., Hans-Filo, G., dos Santos, V., Qaqish, B.F., Rivitti, E.A., Diaz, L.A. 2006. Prevalence of anti-desmoglein-3 antibodies in endemic regions of Fogo Selvagem in Brazil. *J. Invest. Dermatol.* 126, 2044-48.

[178] Sharma, V.K., Prasad, H.R., Khadpur, S., Kumar, A. 2006. Evaluation of desmoglein enzyme-linked immunosorbent assay (ELISA) in Indian patients with pemphigus vulgaris. *Int. J. Dermatol.* 45, 518-22.

[179] Zagrodniuk, I., Weltfried, S., Shtruminger, L., Sprecher, E., Kogan, O., Pollack, S., Bergman, R. 2005. A comparison of anti-desmoglein antibodies and indirect immunofluorescence in the serodiagnosis of pemphigus vulgaris. *Int. J. Dermatol.* 44, 541-54.

[180] Kricheli, D., David, M., Frusic-Zlotkin, M., Goldesmith, D., Rabinov, M., Sulkes, J., Milner, Y. 2000. The distribution of pemphigus vulgaris-IgG subclasses and their reactivity with desmoglein 3 and 1 in pemphigus patients and their first-degree relatives. *Br. J. Dermatol.* 143, 337-342.

[181] Kwon, E.J., Yamagami, J., Nishikawa, T., Amagai, M. 2008. Anti-desmoglein IgG autoantibodies in patients with pemphigus in remission. *J. Eur. Acad. Dermatol. Venereol.* 22, 1070-75.

[182] Patsatsi, A., Kyriakou, A., Giannakou, A., Pavlitou-Tsiontsi, A., Lambropoulos, A., Sotiriadis, D. 2014. Clinical significance of anti-desmoglein-1 and -3 circulating autoantibodies in pemphigus patients measured by area Index and Intensity Score. *Acta Derm. Venereol.* 94, 203-6.

[183] Grando, S.A., Laquer, V.T., Le, H.M. 2011. Sirolimus for acute pemphigus vulgaris: a case report and discussion of dualistic action providing for both immunosuppresion and keratinocyte protection. *J. Am. Acad. Dermatol.* 65, 684-86.

[184] Amagai, M., Ahmed, A.R., Kitajima, Y., Bystryn, J.C., Milner, Y., Gniadecki, R., Hertl, M., Pincelli, C., Fridkis-Hareli, M., Aoyama, Y., Frušič-Zlotkin, M., Müller, E., David, M., Mimouni, D., Vind-Kezunovic, D., Michel, B., Mahoney, M., Grando, S.2006. Are desmoglein autoantibodies essential for the immunopathogenesis of pemphigus vulgaris, or just "witness of disease"? *Exp. Dermatol.* 15, 818-831.

[185] Bohl, K., Natarajan, K., Nagarwalla, N., Mohimen, A., Aoki, V., Ahmed, R. 1995. Correlation of peptide specificity and IgG subclass with pathogenic and nonpathogenic autoantibodies in pemphigus vulgaris: a model for autoimmunity. *Proc. Natl. Acad. Sci. U.S.A.* 92, 5239-43.

[186] Ayatollahi, M., Joubeh, S., Mortazavi, H., Jefferis, R., Ghaderi, A. 2004. IgG4 as the predominant autoantibody in sera from patients with active state of pemphigus vulgaris. *J. Eur. Acad. Dermatol. Venereol.* 18, 221-42.

[187] Warren, S.J.P., Arteaga, L.A., Rivitti, E.A., Aoki, V., Hans-Filho, G., Qaqish, B.F., Lin, M.S., Guidice, G.J., Diaz, L.A. 2003. The role of subclass switching in the pathogenesis of endemic pemphigus foliaceus. *J. Invest. Dermatol.* 120, 104-8.

[188] Bohl, K., Mohimen, A., Ahmed, A.R. 1994. Correlation of subclasses of IgG with disease activity in pemphigus vulgaris. *Dermatology* 189 Suppl 1, 85-89.

[189] Futei, Y., Amagai, M., Ishii, K., Kuroda-Kinoshita, K., Ohya, K., Nishikawa, T. 2001. Predominant IgG 4 subclass in autoantibodies of pemphigus vulgaris and foliaceus. *J. Dermatol. Sci.* 26, 55-61.

[190] Brandsen, R., Frusic-Zlotkin, M., Lyubinov, H., Yunes, F., Michel, B., Tamir, A., Milner, Y., Brenner, S. 1997. Circulating pemphigus IgG in families of patients with

pemphigus: comparison of indirect immunofluorescence, and immunoblotting. *J. Am. Acad. Dermatol.* 36, 44-52.

[191] Jones, C.C., Hamilton, R.G., Jordon, R.E. 1988. Subclass distribution of human IgG autoantibodies in pemphigus. *J. Clin. Immunol.* 8, 43-9.

[192] Torzecka, J.D., Wozniak, K., Kowalewski, C., Waszczykowska, E., Sysa-Jedrzejowska, A., Pac, H.H., Narbutt, J. 2007. Circulating pemphigus autoantibodies in healthy relatives of pemphigus patients: coincidental phenomenon with a risk of disease development? *Arch. Dermatol. Res.* 299, 239-43.

[193] Mentink, L.F., de Jong, M.C., Kloosterhuis, G.J., Zuiderveen, J., Jonkman, M.F., Pas, H.H. 2007. Coexistence of IgA antibodies to desmogleins 1 and 3 in pemphigus vulgaris, pemphigus foliaceus and paraneoplastic pemphigus. *Br. J. Dermatol.* 156, 635-41.

[194] Nagel, A., Lang, A., Engel, D., Podstawa, E., Hunzelmann, N., de Pita, O., Borradori, L., Uter, W., Hertl, M. 2010. Clinical activity of pemphigus vulgaris relates to IgE autoantibodies against desmoglein 3. *Clin. Immunol.* 134, 320-30.

[195] Ohata, Y., Amagai, M., Ishii, K., Hashimoto, T. 2001. Immunoreactivity against intracellular domains of desmogleins in pemphigus. *J. Dermatol. Sci.* 25, 64-71.

[196] Lanza, A., Femiano, F., De Rosa, A., Cammarota, M., Lanza, M., Cirillo, N. 2006. The N-terminal fraction of desmoglein 3 encompassing its immunodominant domain is present in human serum: implications for pemphigus vulgaris autoimmunity. *Int. J. Immunopathol. Pharmacol.* 19, 399-407.

[197] Dmochowski, M., Hashimoto, T., Garrod, D.R., Nishikawa, T. 1993. Desmocollins I and II are recognized by certain sera from patients with various types of pemphigus, particularly Brazilian pemphigus foliaceus. *J. Invest. Dermatol.* 100, 380-84.

[198] Dmochowski, M., Hashimoto, T., Chidgey, M.A., Yue, K.K., Wikinson, R.W., Nishikawa, T., Garrod, D.R.1995. Demonstration of antibodies to bocine desmocollin isoforms in certain pemphigus sera. *Br. J. Dermatol.* 133, 519-25.

[199] Müller, R., Heber, B., Hashimoto, T., Messer, G., Müllegger, R., Niedermeier, A., Hertl, M. 2009. Autoantibodies against desmocollins in European patients with pemphigus. *Clin. Exp. Dermatol.* 34, 898-903.

[200] Hisamatsu, Y., Amagai, M., Garrod, D.R., Kanzaki, T., Hashimoto, T. 2004. The detection of IgG and IgA autoantibodies to desmocollins 1-3 by enzyme-linked immunosorbent assays using baculovirus-expressed proteins, in atypical pemphigus but not in typical pemphigus. *Br. J. Dermatol.* 151, 73-83.

[201] Rafei, D., Müller, R., Ishii, N., Llamazares, M., Hashimoto, T., Hertl, M., Eming, R. 2011. IgG autoantibodies against desmocollin 3 in pemphigus sera induce loss of keratinocyte adhesion. *Am. J. Pathol.* 178, 718-723.

[202] Grando, S.A. 2000. Autoimmunity to keratinocyte acetylcholine receptors in pemphigus. *Dermatology* 201, 290-95.

[203] Beutner, E.H., Jordon, R.E. 1964. Demonstration of skin antibodies in sera of pemphigus vulgaris patients by indirect immunofluorescent staining. *Proc. Soc. Exp. Biol. Med.* 117, 505-10.

[204] Beutner, E.H., Lever, W.F., Witebsky, E., Jordon, R., Chertock, B. 1965. Autoantibodies in pemphigus vulgaris: response to an intercellular substance of epidermis. *JAMA* 192, 682-88.

[205] Van der Wier, G., Pas, H.H., Jonkman, M.F. 2010. Experimental human cell and tissue models of pemphigus. *Dermatol. Res. Pract.* 2010, 14871.

[206] Schiltz, J.R., Michel, B. 1976. Production of epidermal acantholysis in normal human skin *in vitro* by the IgG fraction from pemphigus serum. *J. Invest. Dermatol.* 67, 254-60.

[207] Schlitz, J.R., Michel, B., Papay, R. 1978. Pemphigus antibody interaction with human epidermal cells in culture. *J. Clin. Invest.* 62, 778-88.

[208] Watt, F.M., Mattey, D.L., Garrod, D.R. 1984. Calcium-induced reorganization of desmosomal components in cultured human keratinocytes. *J. Cell. Biol.* 99, 2211-15.

[209] Iwatsuki, K., Sugaya, K., Takigawa, M. 1993. Dynamic expression of pemphigus and desmosomal antigens by cultured keratinocytes. *Br. J. Dermatol.* 128, 16-22.

[210] Denning, M.F., Guy, S.G., Ellerbroek, S.M., Norvell, S.M., Kowalczyk, A.P., Green, K.J.1998. The expression of desmoglein isoforms in cultured human keratinocytes is regulated by calcium, serum, and protein kinase C. *Exp. Cell. Res.* 239, 50-59.

[211] Schmidt, E., Gutberlet, J., Siegmund, D., Berg, D., Wajant, H., Waschke, J. 2009. Apoptosis is not required for acantholysis in pemphigus vulgaris. *Am. J. Physiol. Cell. Physiol.* 296, C162-72.

[212] Cirillo, N., Lanza, M., Femiano, F., Gaeta, G.M., De Rosa, A., Gombos, F., Lanza, A. 2007. If pemphigus vulgaris IgG are the cause of acantholysis, new IgG-independent mechanisms are the concause. *J. Cell. Physiol.* 212, 563-67.

[213] Zillikens, D., Schmidt, E., Reimer, S., Chimanovitch, I., Hardt-Weinelt, K., Rose, C., Bröcker, E.B., Kock, M., Boehncke, W.H. 2001. Antibodies to desmogleins 1 and 3, but not to BP180, induce blisters in human skin grafted onto SCID mice. *J. Pathol.* 193, 117-24.

[214] Rock, B., Martins, C.R., Theofilopoulos, A.N., Balderas, R. S., Anhalt, G.J., Labib, R.S., Futamura, S., Rivitti, E.A., Diaz, L.A. 1989. The pathogenic effect of IgG4 autoantoibodies in endemic pemphigus foliaceus (fogo selvagem). *N. Engl. J. Med.* 320, 1463-69.

[215] Roscoe, J.T., Diaz, L., Sampaio, S.A., Castro, R.M., Labib, R.S., Takahashi, Y., Patel, H., Anhalt, G.J. 1985. Brazilian pemphigus foliaceus autoantibodies are pathogenic to BALB/c mice by passive transfer. *J. Invest. Dermatol.* 85, 538-41.

[216] Amagai, M., Tsunoda, K., Suzuki, H., Nishifuji, K., Koyasu, S., Nishikawa, T. 2000. Use of autoantigen-knockout mice in developing an active autoimmune disease model for pemphigus. *J. Clin. Invest.* 105, 625-31.

[217] Shimizu, A.,Ishiko, A., Ota, T., Tsunoda, K., Koyasu, S., Amagai, M., Nishikawa, T. 2002. Ultrastructural changes in mice actively producing antibodies to desmoglein 3 parallel those in patients with pemphigus vulgaris. *Arch. Dermatol. Res.* 294, 318-23.

[218] Takahashi, H., Amagai, M., Nishikawa, T., Fujii, Y., Kawakami, Y., Kuwana, M. 2008. Novel system evaluating in vivo pathogenicity of desmoglein 3-reactive T cell clones using murine pemphigus vulgaris. *J. Immunol.* 181, 1526-35.

[219] Tsunoda, K., Ota, T., Suzuki, H., Ohyama, M., Nagai, T., Nishikawa, T., Amagai, M., Koyasu, S. 2002. Pathogenic autoantibody production requires loss of tolerance against desmoglein 3 in both T and B cells in experimental pemphigus vulgaris. *Eur. J. Immunol.* 32, 627-33.

[220] Takahashi, Y., Patel, H.P., Labib, R.S., Diaz, L.A., Anhalt, G.J. 1985. Experimentally induced pemphigus vulgaris in neonatal BALB/c mice: a time-course study of clinical,

immunologic, ultrastructural, and cytochemical changes. *J. Invest. Dermatol.* 84, 41-46.

[221] Amagai, M., Hashimoto, T., Shimizu, N., Nishikawa, T. 1994. Absorption of pathogenic autoantibodies by the extracellular domain of pemphigus vulgaris antigen (Dsg3) produced by Baculovirus. *J. Clin. Invest.* 94, 59-67.

[222] Amagai, M., Karpati, S., Prussick, R., Klaus-Kovtun, V., Stanley, J.R. 1992. Autoantibodies against the amino-terminal cadherin-like binding domain of pemphigus vulgaris antigen are pathogenic. *J. Clin. Invest.* 90, 919-26.

[223] Di Zenzo, G., Di Lullo, G., Corti, D., Calabresi, V., Sinistro, A., Vanzetta, F., Didona, B., Cianchini, G., Hertl, M., Eming, R., Amagai, M., Ohyama, B., Hashimoto, T., Sloostra, J., Sallusto, F., Zambruno, G., Lanzavecchia. 2012. Pemphigus autoantibodies generated through somatic mutations target the desmoglein-3 cis-interface. *J. Clin. Invest.* 122, 3781-90.

[224] Shimizu, A., Ishiko, A., Ota, T., Tsunoda, K., Amagai, M., Nishikawa, T. 2004. IgG binds to desmoglein 3 in desmosomes and causes a desmosomal split without keratin retraction in a pemphigus mouse model. *J. Invest. Dermatol.* 122, 1145-53.

[225] Nguyen, V.T., Ndoye, A., Shultz, L.D., Pittelkow, M.R., Grando, S.A. 2000. Antibodies against keratinocyte antigens other than desmogleins 1 and 3 can induce pemphigus vulgaris-like lesions. *J. Clin. Invest.* 106, 1467-79.

[226] Takae, Y., Nishikawa, T., Amagai, M. 2008. Pemphigus mouse model as a tool to evaluate various immunosuppressive therapies. *Exp. Dermatol.* 18, 252-60.

[227] Kalantari-Dehaghi, M., Chen, Y., Deng, W., Chernyavsky, A., Marchenko, S., Wang, P.H., Grando, S.A. 2013. Mechanisms of mitochondrial damage in keratinocytes by pemphigus vulgaris antibodies. *J. Biol. Chem.* 288, 16916-25.

[228] Brickman, C.M., Shoenfeld, Y. 2001. The mosaic of autoimmunity. *Scand. J. Clin. Lab. Invest.* 235 Supp. 3-15.

[229] Bettelli, E., Korn, T., Kuchroo, V.K. 2007. Th17: The third member of the effector T cell trilogy. *Curr. Opin. Immunol.* 19, 652-57.

[230] Martinez, N.E., Sato, F., Kawai, E., Omura, S., Takahashi, S., Yoh, K., Tsunoda, I. 2014. Th 17-biased RORyt transgenic mice become susceptible to a viral model for multiple sclerosis. *Brain. Behav. Immun.* Doi: 10.1016/j.bbi.2014.07.008.

[231] Wu, C., Goodall, J.C., Bush, R., Gaston, J.S. 2014. Relationship of CD146 expression to secretion of interleukin -17, interleukin-22, and interferon-γ by CD4+ T cells in patients with inflammatory arthritis. *Clin. Exp. Immunol.* Doi: 10.1111/cei.12434.

[232] Martin, J.C., Baeten, D.L., Josien, R. 2014. Emerging role of IL-17 and Th17 cells in systemic lupus erythematosus. *Clin. Immunol.* 154, 1-12.

[233] Ha, H.L., Wang, H., Pisitkun, P., Kim, J.C., Tassi, I., Tang, W., Morasso, M.I., Udey, M.C., Siebenlist, U. 2014. IL-17 drives psoriatic inflammation via distinct, target cell-specific mechanisms. *Proc. Natl. Acad. Sci. U.S.A.* 111, e3422-31.

[234] Bettelli, E., Oukka, M., Kuchroo, V.K. 2007. T(H)-17 cells in the circle of immunity and autoimmunity. *Nat. Immunol.* 8, 345-50.

[235] Van der Fits, L., Mourits, S., Voerman, J.S., Kant, M., Boon, L., Laman, J.D., Cornelissen, F., Mus, A.M., Florencia, E., Prens, E.P., Lubberts, E. 2009. Imiquimod-induced psoriasis-like skin inflammation in mice is mediated via the IL-23/IL-17 axis. *J. Immunol.* 182, 5836-45.

[236] Wong, C.K., Lit, L.C., Tam, L.S., Li, E.K., Wong, P.T., Lam, C.W. 2008. Hyperproduction of IL-23 and IL-17 in patients with systemic lupus erythematosus: implications for Th17-mediated inflammation in auto-immunity. *Clin. Immunol.* 127, 385-93.

[237] Yen, D., Cheung, J., Scheerens, H., Poulet, F., McClanahan, T., McKenzie, B., Kleinschek, M.A., Owyang, A., Mattson, J., Blumenschein, W., Murphy, E., Sathe, M., Cua, D.J., Kastelein, R.A., Rennick, D. 2006. IL-23 is essential for T cell-mediated colitis and promotes inflammation via IL-17 and IL-6. *J. Clin. Invest.* 116, 1310-16.

[238] Xue, J., Su, W., Chen, Z., Ke, Y., Du, X., Zhou, Q. 2014. Overexpression of interleukin-23 and interleukin-17 in the lesion of pemphigus vulgaris: a preliminary study. *Mediators Inflamm.* 2014, 463928.

[239] Mauri, C., Bosma, A. 2012. Immune regulatory function of B cells. *Annu Rev. Immunol.* 30, 221-41.

[240] DiLillo, D.J., Matsushita, T., Tedder, T.F. 2010. B10 cells and regulatory B cells balance immune responses during inflammation, autoimmunity, and cancer. *Ann. N Y. Acad. Sci.* 1183, 38-57.

[241] Blair, P.A., Norena, L.Y., Flores-Borja, F., Rawlings, D.J., Isenberg, D.A., Ehrenstein, M.R., Mauri, C. 2010. CD19$^+$CD24^{hi}CD38^{hi} B cells exhibit regulatory capacity in healthy individuals but are functionally impaired in systemic lupus erythematosus patients. *Immunity* 32, 129-140.

[242] Mauri, C., Gray, D., Mushtaq, N., Londei, M. 2003. Prevention of arthritis by interleukin 10-producing B cells. *J. Exp. Med.* 197, 489-501.

[243] Hamel, K.M., Cao, Y., Ashaye, S., Wang, Y., Dunn, R., Kehry, M.R., Glant, T.T., Finnegan, A. 2011. B cell depletion enhances T regulatory cell activity essential in suppression of arthritis. *J. Immunol.* 187, 4900-6.

[244] Knippenberg, S., Peelen, E., Smolders, J., Thewissen, M., Menheere, P., Cohen Tervaert, J.W., Hupperts, R., Damoiseaux, J. 2011. Reduction in IL-10 producing B cells (Breg) in multiple sclerosis is accompanied by a reduced naïve/memory Breg ratio during a relapse but not in remission. *J. Neuroimmunol.* 239, 80-86.

[245] Zha, B., Wang, L., Liu, X., Liu, J., Chen, Z., Xu, J., Sheng, L., Li, Y., Chu, Y. 2012. Decrease in proportion of CD19$^+$ CD24^{hi} CD27$^+$ B cells and impairment of their suppressive function in Graves´ disease. *PloS One* 7, e49835.

[246] Colliou, N., Picard, D., Caillot, F., Calbo, S., Le Corre, S., Lim, A., Lemercier, B., Mauff, B., Maho-Vaillant, M., Jacquot, S., Bedane, C., Bernard, P., Caux, F., Prost, C., Delaporte, E., Doutre, M.S., Dreno, B., Franck, N., Ingen-Housz-Oro, S., Chosidow, O., Pauwels, C., Picard, C., Roujeau, J.C., Sigal, M., Tancrede-Bohin, E., Templier, I., Eming, R., Hertl, M., D´Incan, M., Joly, P., Musette, P. 2013. Long-term remissions of severe pemphigus after rituximab therapy are associated with prolonged failure of desmoglein B cell response. *Sci. Transl. Med.* 175, 175ra30.

[247] Zhu, H.Q., Xu, R.C., Chen, Y.Y., Yuan, H.J., Cao, H., Zhao, X.Q., Zheng, J., Wang, Y., Pan, M. 2014. Impaired function of CD19$^+$ CD24^{hi} CD38^{hi} regulatory B cells in pemphigus patients. *Br. J. Dermatol.* doi: 10.1111/bjd.13192.

[248] Hertl, M., Karr, R., Amagai, M., Katz, S. 1998. Heterogeneous MHC II restriction pattern of autoreactive desmoglein 3 specific T cell responses in pemphigus vulgaris patients and normals. *J. Invest. Dermatol.* 110, 388-92.

[249] Riechers, R., Grötzinger, J., Hertl, M. HLA class II restriction of autoreactive T cells responses in pemphigus vulgaris: review of the literature and potential applications for the development of a specific immunotherapy. *Autoimmunity* 30, 183-96.

[250] Lin, M.S., Swartz, S.J., Lopez, A., Ding, X., Fernandez-Vina, M.A, Stastny, P., Fairley, J.A., Diaz, L.A. 1997. Development and characterization of desmoglein-3 specific T cells from patients with pemphigus vulgaris. *J. Clin. Invest.* 99, 31-40.

[251] Hert, M. 2011. Autoimmune disease of the skin. 3rd revised and enlarged edition. SprigerWienNewYork. 33-59.

[252] Veldman, C., Eming, R., Wolff-Franke, S., Sonderstrup, G., Kwok, W.W., Hertl, M. 2007. Detection of low avidity desmoglein 3-reactive T cells in pemphigus vulgaris using HLA-DRβ1*0402 tetramers. *Clin. Immunol.* 330-37.

[253] Wucherpfennig, K.W., Yu, B., Bhol, K., Monos, D., Argyris, E., Karr, R.W., Ahmed, A.R., Strominger, J.L. 1995. Structural basis for major histocompatibility complex (MHC)-linked susceptibility to autoimmunity: Charged residues of a single MHC binding pocket confer selective presentation of self-peptides in pemphigus vulgaris. *Proc. Natl. Acad. Sci. U.S.A.* 92, 11935-39.

[254] Hertl, M., Eming, R., Veldman, C. 2006. T cell control in autoimmune bullous skin disorders. *J. Clin. Invest.* 116, 1159-66.

[255] Tong, J.C., Tan, T.W., Sinha, A.A., Ranganathan, S.2006. Prediction of desmoglein-3 peptides reveals multiple shared T-cell epitopes in HLA DR4-and DR6-associated pemphigus vulgaris. BMC. *Bioinformatics* 7 (Suppl5), S7.

[256] Nishifuji, K., Amagai, M., Kuwana, M., Iwasaki, T., Nishikawa, T. 2000. Detection of antigen-specific B cells in patients with pemphigus vulgaris by enzyme -linked immunospot assay: requirement of T cell collaboration for autoantibody production. *J. Invest. Dermatol.* 114, 88-94.

[257] Veldman, C., Stauber, A., Wassmuth, R., Uter, W., Schuler, G., Hertl, M. 2003. Dichotomy of autoreactive Th1 and Th2 cell responses to desmoglein 3 in patients with pemphigus vulgaris (PV) and healthy carriers of PV-associated HLA class II alleles. *J. Immunol.* 170, 635-642.

[258] Gebhard KL, Veldman CM, Wassmuth R, Schultz E, Schuler G, Hertl M. 2005. Ex vivo analysis of desmoglein 1-responsive T-helper (Th) 1 and Th2 cells in patients with pemphigus foliaceus and healthy individuals. *Exp. Dermatol.* 14,586-92.

[259] Hertl, M., Amagai, M., Sundaram, H., Stanley, J., Ishii, K., Katz, S.I. 1998. Recognition of desmoglein 3 by autoreactive T cells in pemphigus vulgaris patients and normals. *J. Invest. Dermatol.* 110, 62-66.

[260] Aoki-Ota, M., Kinoshita, M., Ota, T., Tsunoda, K., Iwasaki, T., Tanaka, S., Koyasu, S., Nishikawa, T., Amagai, M. 2006. Tolerance induction by the blockade of CD40/CD154 interaction in pemphigus vulgaris mouse model. *J. Invest. Dermatol.* 126, 105-113.

[261] Noelle, R., Roy, M., Shepherd, D.M., Stamenkovic, I., Ledbetter, J.A, Aruffo, A. 1992. A 39-kDa protein on activated helper T cells binds CD40 and transduces the signal for cognate activation of B cells. *Proc. Natl. Acad. Sci. U.S.A.* 89, 6550-54.

[262] Arakawa, M., Dainichi, T., Yasumoto, S., Hashimoto, T. 2009. Lesional Th17 cells in pemphigus vulgaris and pemphigus foliaceus. *J. Dermatol. Sci.* 53, 228-31.

[263] Djemadji-Oudjiel, N., Goerdt, S., Kodelja, V., Schmuth, M., Orfanos, C.E. 1996. Immunohistochemical identification of type II alternatively activated dendritic

macrophages (RM 3/1+3, MS-1+/-, 25F9-) in psoriatic dermis. *Arch. Dermatol. Res.* 288, 757-64.

[264] Grando, S.A., Glukhensky, B.T., Drannik, G.N., Kostromin, A.P., Boiko, Y. Ya., Senyuk, O.F. 1989. Autoreactive cytotoxic T lymphocytes in pemphigus and pemphigoid. *Autoimmunity* 3, 247-60.

[265] Giurdanella, F., Fania, L., Gnarra, M., Toto, P., Di Rollo, D., Sauder, D.N., Feliciani, C. 2013. A possible role for CD8+ T lymphocytes in the cell-mediated pathogenesis of pemphigus vulgaris. *Mediators Inflamm.* 2013, 764290.

[266] Costantino, C.M., Baecher-Allan, C.M., Hafler, D.A. 2008. Human regulatory T cells and autoimmunity. *Eur. J. Immunol.* 38, 921-24.

[267] Terras, S., Gambicher, T., Moritz, R.K.C., Altmeyer, P., Lambert, J. 2014. Immunohistochemical analysis of FOXP3+ regulatory T cells in healthy human skin and autoimmune dermatoses. *Int. J. Dermatol.* 53, 294-299.

[268] Sugiyama, H., Matsue, H., Nagasaka, A., Nakamura, Y., Tsukamoto, K., Shibagaki, N., Kawamura, T., Kitamura, R., Ando, N., Shimada, S. 2007. CD4+CD25high regulatory T cells are markedly decreased in blood of patients with pemphigus vulgaris. *Dermatology* 214, 210-20.

[269] Veldman, C., Höhne, A., Dieckmann, D., Schuler, G., Hertl, M. 2004. Type I regulatory T cells specific for desmoglein 3 are more frequently detected in healthy individuals than in patients with pemphigus vulgaris. *J. Immunol.* 172, 6468-75.

[270] Thornton, A.M., Shevach, E.M. 2000. Suppressor effector function of CD4$^+$ CD25$^+$ immunoregulatory T cells is antigen nonspecific. *J. Immunol.* 164, 183-90.

[271] Yamaguchi, T., Sakaguchi, S. 2009. Peripheral tolerance to allergen mediated by regulatory T cells. *Nihon Rinsho* 67, 2063-70.

[272] Yamaguchi, T., Sakaguchi, S. 2006. Regulatory T cells in immune surveillance and treatment of cancer. *Semin. Cancer Biol.* 16, 115-23.

[273] Sakaguchi, S., Setoguchi, R., Yagi, H., Nomura, T. 2006. Naturally arising Foxp3-expressing CD25$^+$CD4$^+$ regulatory T cells in self-tolerance and autoimmune disease. *Curr. Top. Microbiol. Immunol.* 305, 51-66.

[274] Sugiyama, H., Matsue, H., Nagasaka, A., Nakamura, Y., Tsukamoto, K., Shibagaki, N., Kawamura, T., Kitamura, R., Ando, N., Shimada, S. 2007. CD4$^+$CD25high regulatory T cells are markedly decreased in blood of patients with pemphigus vulgaris. *Dermatology* 214, 210-20.

[275] Arakawa, M., Dainichi, T., Yasumoto, S., Hashimoto, T. 2009. Lesional Th17 cells in pemphigus vulgaris and pemphigus foliaceus. *J. Dermatol. Sci.* 53, 228-31.

[276] Yokoyama, T., Matsuda, S., Takae, Y., Wada, N., Nishikawa, T., Amagai, M., Koyasu, S. 2011. Antigen-independent development of Foxp3$^+$ regulatory T cells suppressing autoantibody production in experimental pemphigus vulgaris. *Int. Immunol.* 23, 365-73.

[277] Burge, S.M., Wilson, C.L., Dean, D., Wojnarovska, F. 1993. An immunohistological study of desmosomal components in pemphigus. *Br. J. Dermatol.* 128, 363-70.

[278] Kárpáti, S., Amagai, M., Prussick, R., Cehrs, K., Stanley, J.R. 1993. Pemphigus vulgaris antigen, a desmoglein type of cadherin, is localized within keratinocyte desmosomes. *J. Cell Biol.* 122, 409-15.

[279] Amagai, M. 1995. Adhesion molecules. I: Keratinocyte-keratinocyte interactions; cadherins and pemphigus. *J. Invest. Dermatol.* 104, 146-52.

[280] Udey, M.C., Stabley, J.R. 1999. Pemphigus-diseases of antidesmosomal autoimmunity. *JAMA* 282, 572-76.

[281] Amagai, M., Hashimoto, T., Green, K.J., Shimizu, N., Nishikawa, T. 1995. Antigen-specific immunoadsorption of pathogenic autoantibodies in pemphigus foliaceus. *J. Invest. Dermatol.* 104, 895-901.

[282] Bédane, C., Prost, C., Thomine, E., Intrator, L., Joly, P., Caux, F., Blecker, M., Bernard, P., Leboutet, M.J., Tron, F., Lauret, P., Bonnetblanc, J.M., Dubertret, L. 1996. Binding of autoantibodies is not restricted to desmosomes in pemphigus vulgaris: comparison of 14 cases of pemphigus vulgaris and 10 cases of pemphigus foliaceus studied by western immunoblot and immunoelectron microscopy. *Arch. Dermatol. Res.* 288, 343-52.

[283] Waschke, J., Bruggeman, P., Baumgartner, W., Zillikens, D., Drenckhahn. 2005. Pemphigus foliaceus IgG causes dissociation of desmoglein 1-containing junctions without blocking desmoglein 1 transinteraction. *J. Clin. Invest.* 115, 3157-65.

[284] Heupel, W.M., Zillikens, D., Drenckhanh, D., Waschke, J. 2008. Pemphigus vulgaris IgG directly inhibit desmoglein 3-mediated transinteraction. *J. Immunol.* 181, 1825-34.

[285] Müller, E., Williamson, L., Kolly, C., Suter, M.M. 2008. Outside-in signaling through integrins and cadherins: a central mechanism to control epidermal growth and differentiation? *J. Invest. Dermatol.* 128, 501-16.

[286] Sharma, P., Mao, X., Payne, A.S. 2007. Beyond steric hindrance: the role of adhesion signaling pathways in the pathogenesis of pemphigus. *J. Dermatol. Sci.* 48, 1-14.

[287] Bektas, M., Runager, K., Petersen, J.S., Rubenstein, D.S. 2010. Advances in pemphigus research, signaling, and acantholysis. *G. Ital. Dermatol. Venereol.* 145, 675-87.

[288] Kawasaki, Y., Aoyama, Y., Tsunoda, K., Amagai, M., Kitajima, Y. 2006. Pathogenic monoclonal antibody against desmoglein 3 augments desmoglein 3 and p38 MAPK phosphorylation in human squamous carcinoma cell line. *Autoimmunity* 39, 587-90.

[289] Yamamoto, Y., Aoyama, Y., Shu, E., Tsunoda, K., Amagai, M., Kitajima, Y. 2007. Anti-desmoglein 3 (Dsg3) monoclonal antibodies deplete desmosomes of Dsg3 and differ in their Dsg3-depleting activities related to pathogenicity. *J. Biol. Chem.* 282, 17866-76.

[290] Nguyen, B., Dusek, R.L., Beaudry, V.G., Marinkovich, M.P., Attardi, L.D. 2009. Loss of the desmosomal protein Perp enhances the phenotypic effects of pemphigus vulgaris autoantibodies. *J. Invest. Dermatol.* 129, 1710-18.

[291] Caldelari, R., de Bruin, A., Baumann, D., Suter, M.M., Bierkamp, C., Balmer, V., Müller, E. 2001. A central role for the armadillo protein plakoglobin in the autoimmune disease pemphigus vulgaris. *J. Cell Biol.* 153, 823-834.

[292] Grando, S.A., Pittelkow, M.R., Schallreuter, K.U. 2006. Adrenergic and cholinergic control in the biology of epidermis: physiological and clinical significance. *J. Invest. Dermatol.* 126, 1948-65.

[293] Ihrie, R.A., Maeques, M.R., Nguyen, B.T., Horner, J.S., Papazoglu, C., Bronson, R.T., Mills, A.A., Attardi, L.D. 2005. Perp is a p63-regulated gene essential for epithelial integrity. *Cell* 120, 843-856.

[294] Rubenstein, D.S., Diaz, L.A. 2006. Pemphigus antibody induced phosphorylation of keratinocyte proteins. *Autoimmunity* 39, 577-86.

[295] Sánchez-Carpintero, I., Espana, A., Pelacho, B., López Mortalla, N., Rubenstein, D.S., Diaz, L.A., López-Zabalza, M.J. 2004. In vivo blockade of pemphigus vulgaris acantholysis by inhibition of intracellular signal transduction cascades. *Br. J. Dermatol.* 151, 565-70.

[296] Pretel, M., Espana, A., Marquina, M., Pelacho, B., López-Picazo, J.M., López-Zabalza, M.J. 2009. An imbalance in Akt/m TOR is involved in the apoptotic and acantholytic processes in a mouse model of pemphigus vulgaris. *Exp. Dermatol.* 18, 771-80.

[297] Frusic-Zlotkin, M., Raichenberg, D., Wang, X., David, M., Michel, B., Milner, Y. 2006. Apoptotic mechanism in pemphigus autoimmunoglobulins-induced acantholysis -possible involvement of the EGF receptor. *Autoimmunity* 39, 563-75.

[298] Li, X., Ishii, N., Ohata, C., Furumura, M., Hashimoto, T. 2014. Signalling pathways in pemphigus vulgaris. *Exp. Dermatol.* 23, 155-56.

[299] Chernyavsky, A.I., Arredondo, J., Kitajima, Y., Sato-Nagai, M., Grando, S.A. 2007. Desmoglein versus non-desmoglein signaling in pemphigus acantholysis. Characterization of novel signaling pathways downstream of pemphigus vulgaris antigens. *J Biol. Chem.* 282, 13804-12.

[300] Seishima, M., Iwasaki-Bessho, Y., Itoh, Y., Nozawa, Y., Amagai, M., Kitajima, Y. 1999. Phosphatidylcholine-specific phospholipase C, but not phospholipase D, is involved in pemphigus IgG-induced signal transduction. *Arch. Dermatol. Res.* 291, 606-13.

[301] Saito, M., Stahley, S.N., Caughman, C.Y., Mao, X., Tucker, D.K., Payne, A.S., Amagai, M., Kowalczyk, A.P. 2012. Signaling dependent and independent mechanisms in pemphigus vulgaris blister formation. *Plos One* 7, e50696.

[302] Oktarina, D.A., van der Wier, G., Diercks, G.F., Jonkman, M.F., Pas, H.H. 2011. IgG-induced clustering of desmogleins 1 and 3 in skin of patients with pemphigus fits with the desmoglein nonassembly depletion hypothesis. *Br. J. Dermatol.* 165, 552-62.

[303] Calkins, C.C., Setzer, S.V., Jennings, J.M., Summers, S., Tsunoda, K., Amagai, M., Kowalczyk, A.P. 2006. Desmoglein endocytosis and desmosome disassembly are coordinated responses to pemphigus autoantibodies. *J. Biol. Chem.* 281, 7623-34.

[304] Delva, E., Jenning, J.M., Calkins, C.C., Kottke, M.D., Faundez, V., Kowalczyk, A.P. 2008. Pemphigus vulgaris IgG-induced desmoglein-3 endocytosis and desmosomal disassembly are mediated by a clathrin-and dynamin-independent mechanism. *J. Biol. Chem.* 283-18303-13.

[305] Pike, L.J. 2006. Rafts defined: a report on the Keystone symposium on lipid rafts and cell function. *J. Lipid Res.* 47, 1597-98.

[306] Stahley, S.N., Saito, M., Faundez, V., Koval, M., Mattheyses, A.L., Kowalczyk, A.P. 2014. Desmosome assembly and disassembly are membrane raft-dependent. *Plos One* 9, e87809.

[307] de Bruin, A., Calderani, R., Williamson, L., Suter, M.M., Hunziker, T., Wyder, M., Müller, E.J. 2007. Plakoglobin-dependent disruption of the desmosomal plaque in pemphigus vulgaris. *Exp. Dermatol.*16, 468-75.

[308] Galichet, A., Borradori, L., Müller, E.J. 2014. A new light on an old disease: adhesion signaling in pemphigus vulgaris. *J. Invest. Dermatol.* 134, 8-10.

[309] Mao, X., Sano, Y., Park, J.M., Payne, A.S. 2011. p38 MAPK activation is downstream of the loss of intercellular adhesion in pemphigus vulgaris. *Biol. Chem.* 286, 1283-91.

[310] Müller, E.J., Hunziker, T., Suter, M.M. 2007. Keratin intermediate filament retraction is linked to plakoglobin-dependent signaling in pemphigus vulgaris. *J. Am. Acad. Dermatol.* 56, 890-91.

[311] Baroni, A., Buommino, E., Paoletti I, Orlando M, Ruocco E, Ruocco V. 2004. Pemphigus serum and captopril induce heat shock protein 70 and inducible nitric oxide synthase overexpression, triggering apoptosis in human keratinocytes. *Br. J. Dermatol.* 150, 1070-80.

[312] Diercks, G.F., Pas, H.H., Jonkman, M.F. 2009. The utrastructure of acantholysis in pemphigus vulgaris. *Br. J. Dermatol.* 160, 460-61.

[313] Sams, W.M. Jr, Gammon, W.R. 1982. Mechanism of lesion production in pemphigus and pemphigoid. *J. Am. Acad. Dermatol.* 6, 431-52.

[314] Bystryn, J.C., Grando, A. 2006. A novel explanation for acantholysis in pemphigus vulgaris: the basal cell shrinkage hypothesis. *J. Am. Acad. Dermatol.* 54, 513-16.

[315] Gera, J.F., Mellinghoff, I.K., Shi, Y., Rettig, M.B., Tran, C., Hsu, J., Sawyers, C.L., Lichtenstein, A.K. 2004. AKT activity determines sensitivity to mammalian target of rapamycin (mTOR) inhibitors by regulating cyclin D1 and c-myc expression. *J. Biol. Chem.* 279, 2737-46.

[316] Gorshtein, A., Rubinfeld, H., Kendler, E., Theodoropoulou, M., Cerovac, V., Stalla, G.K., Cohen, Z.R., Hadani, M., Shimon, I. 2009. Mammalian target of rapamycin inhibitors rapamycin and RAD001 (everolimus) induce anti-proliferative effects in GH-secreting pituitary tumor cells in vitro. *Endocr. Relat. Cancer.* 16, 1017-27.

[317] Arredondo, J., Chernyavsky, I., Karaouni, A., Grando, S.A. 2005. Novel mechanism of target cell death and survival and of therapeutic action of IVIG in pemphigus. *Am. J. Pathol.*167, 1531-44.

[318] Hengartner, M.O. 2000. The biochemistry of apoptosis. *Nature* 407, 770-6.

[319] Wang, X., Brégégére, F., Frusic-Zlotkin, M., Feinmesser, M., Michel, B., Milner, Y. 2004. Possible apoptotic mechanism in epidermal cell acantholysis induced by pemphigus vulgaris autoimmunoglobulins. *Apotosis* 9, 131-43.

[320] Zuccolotto, I., Rosellino, A.M., Ramalho, L.N., Zucoloto, S. 2003. Apoptosis and p63 expression in the pathogenesis of bullous lesions of endemic pemphigus foliaceus. *Arch. Dermatol. Res.* 295, 284-86.

[321] Puviani, M., Marconi, A., Cozzani, E., Pincelli, C. 2003. Fas ligand in pemphigus sera induces keratinocyte apoptosis through the activation of caspase-8. *J. Invest. Dermatol.* 120, 164-67.

[322] Rodrigues, D.B., Pereira, S.A., dos Reis, M.A., Adad, S.J., Caixeta, J.E., Chiba, A.M., Sousa, R.A., Rodrigues, V. Jr. 2009. In situ detection of inflammatory cytokines and apoptosis in pemphigus foliaceus patients. *Arch. Pathol. Lab. Med.* 133, 97-100.

[323] Lyndsay, D., Gray, D., Soiller, D., White, M.R, Damato, B., Grierson, I., Paraoan, L. 2009. P53 apoptosis mediator PERP: localization, function and caspase activation in uveal melanoma. *J. Cell. Mol. Med.* 13, 1995-2007.

[324] Grando, S.A. Decompensation in proteinase-inhibitor system and application of proteinase inhibitors in pemphigus and pemphigoid. *J. Dermatol. Sci.* 4, 95-97.

[325] Pacheco-Tovar, M.G., Avalos-Diaz, E., Vega-Memije, E., Bollain-y-Goytia, J.J., López-Robles, E., Hoiyo-Tomoka, M.T., Domínquez-Soto, L., Herrera-Esparza, R. 2009. The final destiny of acantholytic cells in pemphigus is Fas mediated. *J. Eur. Acad. Dermatol. Venereol.* 23, 697-701.

[326] Grando, S.A., Glukhenky, B.T., Drannik, G.N., Epshtein, E.V., Kostromin, A.P., Korostash, T.A. 1989. Mediators of inflammation in blister fluids from patients with pemphigus vulgaris and bullous pemphigoid. *Arch. Dermatol.* 125, 925-30.

[327] Rico, M.J. Benning, C., Weingart, E.S., Streilein, R.D., Hall, R.P.1999. Characterization of skin cytokines in bullous pemphigoid and pemphigus vulgaris. *Br. J. Dermatol.* 140, 1079-86.

[328] Grando, S.A., Bystryn, J.C., Chernyavsky, A., Frušic-Zlotkin, M., Gniadecki, R., Lotti, R., Milner, Y., Pittelkow, M.R., Pincelli, C.2009. Apoptolysis: a novel mechanism of skin blistering in pemphigus vulgaris linking the apoptotic pathways to basal shrinkage and suprabasal acantholysis. *Exp. Dermatol.* 18, 764-770.

[329] Jolly, P.S., Berkowitz, P., Bektas, M., Lee, H.E., Chua, M., Diaz, L.A., Rubenstein, D.S. p38 MAPK signaling and desmoglein-3 internalization are linked event in pemphigus acantholysis. *J. Biol. Chem.* 285, 8936-41.

[330] Chernyavsky, A.I., Arrendo, J., Piser, T., Karlsson, E., Grando, S.A. 2008. Differential coupling of M_1muscarinic and $\alpha 7$ nicotinic receptors to inhibition of pemphigus acantholysis. *J. Biol. Chem.* 283, 3401-8.

[331] Berkowitz, P., Hu, P., Warren, S., Liu, Z., Diaz, L., Rubenstein, D.S. 2006. p38MAPK inhibition prevents disease in pemphigus vulgaris mice. *Proc. Natl. Acad. Sci. U.S.A.* 103, 12855-60.

[332] Mavropoulos, A., Orfanidou, T., Liaskos, C., Smyk, D.S., Spyrou, V., Sakkas, L., Rigopoulou, E.I., Bogdanos, D.P. 2013. p38 MAPK signaling in pemphigus: implications for skin autoimmunity. *Autoimmune Dis.* 2013, 728859.

[333] Waschke, J., Spindler, V. 2014. Desmosomes and extradesmosomal adhesive signaling contacts in pemphigus. *Med. Res. Rev.* 34. 1127-45.

[334] Lanza, A., Cirillo, N. 2006. Caspase-dependent cleavage of desmoglein 1 depends on the apoptotic stimulus. *Br. J. Dermatol.* 156, 378-410.

[335] Cirillo, N., Lanza, M., De Rosa, A., Cammarota, M., La Gatta, A., Gombos, F., Lanza, A. 2008. The most widespread desmosomal cadherin, desmoglein 2, is a novel target of caspase 3-mediated apoptotic machinery. *J. Cell. Biochem.* 103, 598-606.

[336] Wilgram, G.F., Caufield, J.B., Lever, W.F. 1964. Electron microscopic studies in skin diseases with acantholysis (pemphigus vulgaris, pemphigus familiaris benignus chronicus, Darier´disease). *Dermatol. Wochenschr.* 147, 281-92.

[337] Hu, C.H., Beno, M., Schiltz, J.R. 1978. Epidermal acantholysis induced *in vitro* by pemphigus autoantibody. *Am. J. Pathol.* 90, 345-62.

[338] Weiske, J., Schöneberg, T., Schröder, W., Hatzfeld, M., Tauber, R., Huber, O. 2001. The fate of desmosomal proteins in apoptotic cells. *J. Biol. Chem.* 276, 41175-81.

[339] Dusek, R.L., Getsios, S., Chen, F., Park, J.K., Amargo, E.V., Cryns, V.L., Green, K.J. 2006. The differentiation-dependent desmosomal cadherin desmoglein 1 is a novel caspase-3 target that regulates apoptosis in keratinocytes. *J. Biol. Chem.* 281, 3614-24.

[340] Caulín, C., Salvesen, G.S., Oshima, R.G. 1997. Caspase cleavage of keratin 18 and reorganization of intermediate filaments during epithelial cell apoptosis. *J. Cell. Biol.* 138, 1379-94.

[341] Steinhusen, U., Badock, V., Bauert, A., Behrens, J., Liebold, B.W., Dörken, B., Bommert, K. 2000. Apoptosis-induced cleavage of β-catenin by caspase-3 results in proteolytic fragments with reduced transactivation potential. *J. Biol. Chem.* 275, 16345-53.

[342] Nguyen, V.T., Arredondo, J., Chernyavsky, A.I., Pittelkov, M.R., Kitajima, Y., Grando, S.A. 2004. Pemphigus vulgaris acantholysis ameliorated by cholinergic agonists. *Arch. Dermatol.* 140, 327-334.

[343] Aoyama, Y., Owada, M.K., Kitajima, Y. 1999. A pathogenic autoantibody, pemphigus vulgaris-IgG induces phosphorylation of desmoglein 3, and its dissociation from plakoglobin in cultured keratinocytes. *Eur. J. Immunol.* 29, 2233-40.

[344] Gilbert, S., Loranger, A., Daigle, N., Marceau, N. 2001. Simple epithelium keratins 8 and 18 provide resistance to FAS-mediated apoptosis. The protection occurs through a receptor-targeting modulation. *J. Cell Biol.* 154, 763-73.

[345] Inada, H., Izawa, I., Nishizawa, M., Fujita, E., Kiyono, T., Takahashi, T., Momoi, T., Inagaki, M. 2001. Keratin attenuates tumor necrosis factor-induced cytotoxicity through association with TRADD. *J. Cell Biol.* 155, 415-425.

[346] Lanza, A., Cirillo, N., Rossiello, R., Rienzo, M., Cuttilo, L., Casamassimi, A., de Nigris, F., Schiano, C., Rossiello, L., Femiamo, F., Gombos, F. 2008. Evidence of key role of Cdk2 overexpression in pemphigus vulgaris. *J. Biol. Chem.* 283, 8736-45.

[347] Baccarelli, A., Wright, R.O., Bollati, V., Tarantini, L., Litonjua, A.A., Suh, H.H., Zanobetti, A., Sparrow, D., Vokonas, P.S., Schwartz, J. 2009. Rapid DNA methylation changes after exposure to traffic particles. *Am. J. Respir. Crit. Care Med.* 179, 572-578.

[348] Vojdani, A. 2014. A potential link between environmental triggers and autoimmunity. *Autoimmune Dis.* 2014, 437231.

[349] Brenner, S., Tur, E., Shapiro, J., Ruocco, V., D´Avino, M., Ruocco, E., Tsankov, N., Vassileva, S., Drenovska, K., Brezoev, P., Barnadas, M.A., Gonzales, M.J., Anhalt, G., Nousari, H., Silva, M.R., Pinto, T.P., Miranda, M.F. 2001. Pemphigus vulgaris: environmental factors. Occupational, behavioral, medical, and qualitative food frequency. *Int. J. Dermatol.* 40, 562-69.

[350] Ruocco, V., Ruocco, E. 2003. Pemphigus and environmental factors. *G. Ital. Dermatol. Venereol.* 138, 299-309.

[351] Ruocco, V., Ruocco, E., Lo Schiavo, A., Brunetti, G., Guerrera, L.P., Wolf, R. 2013. Pemphigus: Etiology, pathogenesis, and inducing or triggering factors? Facts and controversies. *Clin. Dermatol.* 31, 374-381.

[352] Yokel, B.K., Hood, A.F., Anhalt, G.J. 1989. Induction of acantholysis in organ explants culture by penicillamine and captopril. *Arch. Dermatol.* 125, 1367-70.

[353] Yanagishita, T., Tamada, Y., Watanabe, D. 2014. Bucillamine-induced pemphigus vulgaris. *J. Eur. Acad. Dermatol. Venereol.* doi 10.1111/jdv.12472.

[354] Hur, J.W., Lee, C.W., Yoo, D.H. 2006. Bucillamine-induced pemphigus vulgaris in a patient with rheumatoid arthritis and polymyositis overlap syndrome. *J. Korean Med. Sci.* 21, 585-87.

[355] Ogata, K., Nakajima, H., Ikeda, M., Yamamoto, Y., Amagai, M., Hashimoto, T., Kodama, H. 2001. Drug-induced pemphigus foliaceus with features of pemphigus vulgaris. *Br. J. Dermatol.* 144, 421-22.

[356] Fujita, H., Iguchi, M., Watanabe, R., Asahina, A. 2007. Pemphigus foliaceus induced by bucillamine. *Eur. J. Dermatol.* 17, 98-99.

[357] Ogawa, H., Taneda, A., Kanaoka, Y., Sekine, T. 1979. The histochemical distribution of protein bound sulfhydryl groups in human epidermis by the new staining method. *J. Histochem. Cytochem.* 27, 942-46.

[358] Brenner, S., Goldber, I. 2011. Drug-induced pemphigus. *Clin. Dermatol.* 29, 455-57.

[359] Newby, C.S., Barr, R.M., Greaves, M.W., Mallet, A. 2000. Cytokine release and cytotoxicity in human keratinocytes and fibroblasts induced by phenols and sodium dodecyl sulfate. *J. Invest. Dermatol.* 115, 292-98.

[360] Brenner, S., Ruocco, V., Ruocco, E., Srebrnik, A., Goldberg, I. 2006. A possible mechanism for phenol-induced pemphigus. *Skinmed* 5, 25-26.

[361] Tsankov, N., Dimitrowa, J., Obreschkowa, E., Lasarowa, A. 1987. Induced pemphigus by the pesticide phosphamide. *Z. Hautkr.* 62, 196-201.

[362] Ruocco, V., De Angelis, E., Lombardi, M.L. 1993. Drug-induced pemphigus. II. Pathomechanisms and experimental investigations. *Clin. Dermatol.* 11, 507-13.

[363] Wolf, R., Brenner, S. 1994. An active amide group in the molecule of drugs that induce pemphigus: a casual or casual relationship. *Dermatology* 189, 1-4.

[364] Anadolu, R.Y., Birol, A., Bostanci, S., Boyvat, A. 2002. A case of pemphigus vulgaris possibly triggered by quinolones. *J. Eur. Acad. Dermatol. Venereol.* 16, 152-153.

[365] Valeyrie-Allanore, L., Sassolas, B., Roujeau, J.C. 2007. Drug-induced skin, nail and hair disorders. *Drug. Saf.* 30, 1011-30.

[366] Kivity, S., Agmon-Levin, N., Blank, M., Shoenfeld, Y. 2009. Infection and autoimmunity-friends or foes? *Trends. Immunol.* 30, 409-14.

[367] Sagi, L., Sherer, Y., Trau, H., Shoenfeld, Y. 2008. Pemphigus and infectious agents. *Autoimmun. Rev.* 8, 33-35.

[368] Sagi, L., Baum, S., Agmon-Levin, N., Sherer, Y., Katz, B.S., Barzilai, O., Ram, M., Bizzaro, N., SanMarco, M., Trau, H., Shoenfeld, Y. 2011. Autoimmune bullous diseases. The spectrum of infectious agent antibodies and review of the literature. *Autoimmun. Rev.* 10, 527-535.

[369] Caldarola, G., Kneisel, A., Hertl, M., Feliciani, C. 2008. Herpes simplex virus infection in pemphigus vulgaris: clinical and immunological considerations. *Eur. J. Dermatol.* 18, 440-43.

[370] Kalra, A., Ratho, R.K. 2005. Role of herpes simplex and cytomegalo viruses in recalcitrant oral lesions of pemphigus vulgaris. *Int. J. Dermatol.* 44, 259-260.

[371] Senger, P., Sinha, A.A. 2012. Exploring the link between herpes viruses and pemphigus vulgaris: literature review and commentary. *Eur. J. Dermatol.* 22, 728-35.

[372] Esmaili, N., Hallaji, Z., Abedini, R., Soori, T., Mortazavi, H., Chams-Davatchi, C. 2010. Pemphigus vulgaris and herpes viruses: is there any relationship? *Int. J. Dermatol.* 49, 1261-65.

[373] Kurata, M., Mizukawa, Y., Aoyma, Y., Shiohara, T. 2014. Herpes simplex virus reaction as a trigger of mucous lesions in pemphigus vulgaris. *Br. J. Dermatol.* 171, 554-60.

[374] Oliviera-Batista, D.P., Janini, M.E., Fernandes, N.C., Santos, N. 2013. Laboratory diagnosis of herpesvirus infections in patients with pemphigus vulgaris lesions. *Intervirology.* 56, 231-36.

[375] Gye, J., Nan, C.H., Kim, J.S., Kim, J.Y., Park, B.C., Kim, M.H., Hong, S.P. 2014. Pemphigus vulgaris in pregnancy associated with herpes virus type I infection. *Ann. Dermatol.* 26, 258-60.

[376] Memar, O.M., Rady, P.L., Goldblum, R.M., Yen, A., Tyring, S.K. 1997. Human herpesvirus 8 DNA sequences in blistering skin from patients with pemphigus. *Arch. Dermatol.* 133, 1247-51.

[377] Bezold, G., Sander, C.A., Flaid, M.J., Peter, R.U., Messer, G. 2000. Lack of detection of human herpesvirus (HHV)-8 DNA in lesional skin of German pemphigus vulgaris and pemphigus foliaceus patients. *J. Invest. Dermatol.* 114, 739-41.

[378] Markitzu, A., Pisanty, S. 1993. Pemphigus vulgaris after infection by Epstein-Bar virus. *Int. J. Dermatol.* 32, 917-18.

[379] Barzilai, O., Sherer, Y., Ram, M., Izhaky, D., Anaya, J.M., Shoenfeld, Y. 2007. Epstein-Bar virus and cytomegalovirus in autoimmune disease: are they truly notorious? A preliminary report. *Ann. N.Y. Acad. Sci.* 1108, 567-77.

[380] Stevenson, M.L., Levitt, J.O. 2011. Acute zoster in known pemphigus vulgaris and bullous pemphigoid: avoiding the" disease flare" trap. *J. Am. Acad. Dermatol.* 64, e125-26.

[381] Sinha, P., Chatterjee, M., Vasudevan, B. 2014. Pemphigus vulgaris: a dermatological sequel of severe H1N1 infection. *Indian Dermatol. Online* J.5, 216-17.

[382] Goon, A.T., Tay, Y.K., Tan, S.H. 2001. Pemphigus vulgaris following varicella infection. *Clin. Exp. Dermatol.* 26, 661-63.

[383] Demerci, G.T., Mansur, A.T., Altunay, I.K., Aydingoz, I.E., Atis, G. 2014. Hepatitis C and hepatitis B virus infections in the etiopathogenesis of pemphigus. *An. Bras. Dermatol.* 89, 423-26.

[384] Brenner, S., Sasson, A., Sharon, O. 2002. Pemphigus and infections. *Clin. Dermatol.* 20, 114-18.

[385] Leshem, Y.A., Gdalevich, M., Ziv, M., David, M., Hodak, E., Mimouni, D. 2014. Opportunistic infections in patients with pemphigus. *J. Am. Acad. Dermatol.* 71, 284-92.

[386] Amagai, M., Matsuyoshi, N., Wang, Z.H., Andl, C., Stanley, J.R. 2000. Toxin in bullous impetigo and staphylococcal scalded-skin syndrome targets desmoglein 1. *Nat. Med.* 11, 1275-77.

[387] Amagai, M. 2003. Desmoglein as a target in autoimmunity and infection. *J. Am. Acad. Dermatol.* 48, 244-52.

[388] Ruocco, V., Vitale, O., Astarita, C. 1980. Transient pemphigus induced by sunburn. *J. Cutan. Pathol.* 7, 429-30.

[389] Maramatsu, T., Iida, T., Ko, T., Shirai, T. 1996. Pemphigus vulgaris exacerbated by exposure to sunlight. *J. Dermatol.* 23, 559-63.

[390] Aghassi, D., Dover, J.S. 1998. Pemphigus foliaceus induced by psoralen-UV-A. *Arch. Dermatol.* 134, 1300-1.

[391] Kano, Y., Shimosegawa, M., Mizukawa, Y., Shiohara, T. 2000. Pemphigus foliaceus induced by exposure to sunlight. Report of a case and analysis of photochallenge-induced lesions. *Dermatology* 201,132-38.

[392] Orion, E., Matz, H., Wolf, R. 2004. Pemphigus vulgaris induced by radiotherapy. *J. Eur. Acad. Dermatol. Venereol.* 18, 508-9.

[393] Ambay, A., Stratman, E. 2006. Ionizing radiation-induced pemphigus foliaceus. *J. Am. Acad. Dermatol.* 54, S251-52.

[394] Fried, R., Lynfield, Y., Vitale, P., Anhalt, G. 1993. Paraneoplastic pemphigus appearing as bullous pemphigoid-like eruption after palliative radiation therapy. *J. Am. Acad. Dermatol.* 29, 815-17.

[395] Robbins, A., Lazarova, Z., Janson, M.M., Fairley, J.A. 2007. Pemphigus vulgaris presenting in a radiation portal. *J. Am. Acad. Dermatol.* 56, S82-85.

[396] Delaporte, E., Piette, F., Bergoend, H. 1991. Pemphigus vulgaris induced by radiotherapy. *Ann. Dermatol. Venereol.* 118, 447-51.

[397] Low, G.J., Keelling, J.H. 1990. Ionizing radiation-induced pemphigus. Case presentations and literature review. *Arch. Dermatol.* 126, 1319-23.

[398] Tan, S.R, McDermott, M.R., Castillo, C.J., Sauder, D.N. 2006. Pemphigus vulgaris induced by electrical injury. *Cutis* 77, 161-65.

[399] Vignale, R., Espasandin, J., Cassinelli, A., Cassella de Vilaboa, E., Gonzales, V.1993. Pemphigus vulgaris after electrosurgery (thermal-heat therapy) of a basal cell carcinoma. *Int. J. Dermatol.* 32, 307-8.

[400] Tsankov, N., Stransky, L., Kostowa, M., Mitrowa, T., Obreschkowa, E. 1990. Induced pemphigus caused by occupational contact with basochrom. *Derm. Beruf. Umwelt.* 38, 91-93.

[401] Tsankov, N., Kazadjieva, J., Gantcheva, M. 1998. Contact pemphigus induced b dihydrodiphenyltrichloethane. *Eur. J. Dermatol.* 8, 42-43.

[402] Goldberg, I., Kashman, Y., Brenner, S. 1999. The induction of pemphigus by phenol drugs. *Int. J. Dermatol.* 38, 888-92.

[403] Lambert, J., Schepens, P., Janssens, J., Dockx P. 1986. Skin lesions as a sign of subacute pentachlorophenol intoxication. *Acta Derm. Venereol.* 66, 170-72.

[404] Kaplan, R.P., Detwiler, S.P., Saperstein, H.W. 1993. Physically induced pemphigus after cosmetic procedures. *Int. J. Dermatol.* 32, 100-3.

[405] Brenner, S., Srebrnik, A., Goldberg, I. 2004. Pemphigus can be induced by topical phenol as well as by foods and drugs that contain phenols or thiols. *J. Cosmet. Dermatol.* 2, 161-65.

[406] Brenner, S., Ruocco, V., Wolf, R., de Angelis, E., Lombardi, M.L. 1995. Pemphigus and dietary factors. In vitro acantholysis by allyl compounds of genus Allium. *Dermatology* 190, 197-202.

[407] Feliciani, C., Ruocco, E,, Zampetti, A., Toto, P., Amerio, P., Tulli, A., Amerio, P., Ruocco, V. 2007. Tannic acid induces in vitro acantholysis of keratinocytes via IL-1α and TNF-α. *Int. J. Immunopathol. Pharmacol.* 20, 289-99.

[408] Ruocco,V., Brenner, S., Ruocco, E. 2001. Pemphigus and diet: does a link exist? *Int. J. Dermatol.* 40, 161-63.

[409] Tur, E., Brenner, S. 1997. Contributing exogenous factors in pemphigus. *Int. J. Dermatol.* 36, 888-93.

[410] Stojanovich, L. 2010. Stress and autoimmunity. *Autoimmun. Rev.* 9, A271-76.

[411] Morell-Dubois, S., Carpentier, O., Cottencin, O., Queyrel, V., Hachulla, E., Hantron, P.Y., Delaporte, E. 2008. Stressful life events and pemphigus. *Dermatology* 216, 104-8.

[412] Mehta, J.N., Martin, A.G. 2000. A case of pemphigus vulgaris improved by cigarette smoking. *Arch. Dermatol.* 136, 15-17.

[413] Grando, S.A., Dahl, M.V. 2000. Nicotine and pemphigus. *Arch. Dermatol.* 136, 1269.

[414] Mignogna, M.D., Lo Muzio, L., Ruocco, E. 2000. Pemphigus induction by influenza vaccination. *Int. J. Dermatol.* 39, 800.

[415] Cozzani, E., Cacciapuoti, M., Parodi, A., Rebora, A. 2002. Pemphigus following tetanus and diphtheria vaccination. *Br. J. Dermatol.* 147, 188-89.

[416] Berkun, Y., Mimouni, D., Shoenfeld, Y. 2005. Pemphigus following hepatitis B vaccination--coincidence or causality? *Autoimmunity* 38, 117-19.

[417] Yalcin, B., Alli, N. 2007. Pemphigus vulgaris following antirabies vaccination. *J. Dermatol.* 34, 734-35.

[418] Kavusi, S., Daneshpazhooh, M., Farahani F., Abedini, R., Lajevardi, V., Chams-Davatchi, C. 2008. Outcome of pemphigus vulgaris. *J. Eur. Acad. Dermatol. Venereol.* 22, 580-84.

[419] Saha, M., Bhogal, B., Black, M.M., Cooper, D., Vaughan, R.W., Groves, R.W. 2014. Prognostic factors in pemphigus vulgaris and pemphigus foliaceus. *Br. J. Dermatol.* 170, 116-22.

[420] Harman, K.E., Gratian, M.J., Bhogal, B.S., Challacombe, S.J., Black, M.M. 2000. A study of desmoglein 1 autoantibodies in pemphigus vulgaris: racial differences in frequency and the association with a more severe phenotype. *Br. J. Dermatol.* 143, 343-48.

[421] Herrero-Gonzales, J.E., Iranzo, P., Benítez, D., Lozano, F., Herrero, C. 2010. Correlation of immunological profile with phenotype and disease outcome in pemphigus. *Acta Derm. Venereol.* 90, 401-5.

[422] Iraji, F., Yoopsefi, A. 2006. Healing effect of Pilocarpine gel 4% on skin lesions of pemphigus vulgaris. *Int. J. Dermatol.* 45, 743-46.

[423] Chaffins, M.L., Collins, D., Fivenson, D.P. 1993. Treatment of pemphigus and linear IgA dermatosis with nicotinamide and tetracycline: a review of 13 cases. *J. Am. Acad. Dermatol.* 28, 998-1000.

[424] Valikhani, M., Kavusi, S., Chams-Davatchi, C., Hallaji, Z., Esmaili, N., Ghandi, N., Farahani, F., Lajevardi, V. 2008. Impact of smoking on pemphigus. *Int. J. Dermatol.* 47, 567-70.

[425] Shimizu, H., Masunaga, T., Ishiko, A., Kikuchi, A., Hashimoto, T., Nishikawa, T. 1995. Pemphigus vulgaris and pemphigus foliaceus sera show an inversely graded binding pattern to extracellular regions of desmosomes in different layers of human epidermis. *J. Invest. Dermatol.* 105, 153-59.

[426] Švecová D. 2014. Handbook of dermatovenerology for practical lessons. 2nd Edition. Comenius University. Bratislava, 45-55.

[427] Vaughn Jones, S.A., Palmer, I., Bhogal, B.S., Eady, R.A., Black, M.M. 1995. The use of Michel´s transport medium for immunofluorescence and immunoelectron microscopy in autoimmune bullous diseases. *J. Cutan. Pathol.* 22, 365-70.

[428] Abreu Velez, A.M., Calle, J., Howard, M.S. 2013. Autoimmune epidermal blistering diseases. *Our Dermatol. Online* 4 (Suppl.3), 631-46.

[429] Radoš, J. 2011. Autoimmune blistering diseases: histologic meaning. *Clin. Dermatol.* 29, 377-88.

[430] Baum, S., Sakka, N., Artsi, O., Trau, H., Barzilai, A. 2014. Diagnosis and classification of autoimmune blistering diseases. *Autoimmun. Rev.* 13, 482-89.

[431] Kershenovich, R., Hodak, E., Mimouni, D. 2014. Diagnosis and classification of pemphigus and bullous pemphigoid. *Autoimmun. Rev.* 13, 477-81.

[432] Ruocco, V., Ruocco, E. 1999. Tzank smear, an old test for the new millennium: when and how. *Int. J. Dermatol.* 38, 830-34.

[433] Ruocco, E., Brunetti, G., Del Vecchio, M., Ruocco, V. 2011. The practical use of cytology for diagnosis in dermatology. *J. Eur. Acad. Dermatol. Venereol.* 25, 125-29.

[434] Beutner, E.H., Lever, W.F., Witebsky, E., Jordon, R,, Chertock, B. 1965. Autoantibodies in pemphigus vulgaris: response to an intercellular substance of epidermis. *JAMA* 192, 682-88.

[435] Schmidt, E., Zillikens. D. 2010. Modern diagnosis of autoimmune blistering skin diseases. *Autoimmun. Rev.* 10, 84-89.

[436] Kneisel, A., Hertl, M. 2011. Autoimmune bullous skin diseases. Part 2: diagnosis and therapy. *J. Dtsch. Dermatol. Ges.* 11, 927-47.

[437] Ko, C.J., McNiff, J.M. 2014. Punctate pemphigus: an underreported direct immunofluorescence pattern. *J. Cutan. Pathol.* 41, 293-96.

[438] Harrist, T.J., Mihn, M.C. 1979. Cutaneous immunopathology. The diagnostic use of direct and indirect immunofluorescence techniques in dermatologic disease. *Hum. Pathol.*10, 625-53.

[439] Zhong, S., Qiu, Y.F., Han, B.B., Zhao, J.Y., Zhu, X.J., Chen, X.X. 2011. Detection of serum desmoglein antibody level using enzyme-linked immunosorbent assay (ELISA) for monitoring disease activity in patients with pemphigus vulgaris. *Beijing Da Yue Xue Bao.* 43, 414-15.

[440] Harman, K.E., Gratian, M.J., Seed, P.T., Bhogal, B.S., Challacombe, S.J., Black, M,M. 2000. Diagnosis of pemphigus by ELISA: a critical evaluation of two ELISAs for detection of antibodies to the major pemphigus antigens. *Clin. Exp. Dermatol.* 25, 236-40.

[441] Tampoia, M., Giavarina, D., Di Giorgo, C., Bizzaro, N. 2012. Diagnostic accuracy of enzyme-linked immunosorbent assay (ELISA) to detect anti-skin autoantibodies in autoimmune blistering skin disease: a systemic review and meta-analysis. *Autoimmun. Rev.* 12, 121-26.

[442] Balighi, K., Taheri, A., Mansoori, P., Champs, C. 2006. Value of direct immunofluorescence in predicting remission in pemphigus vulgaris. *Int. J. Dermatol.* 45, 1308-11.

[443] Švecová, D. 2009. Pemphigus. Bonus, Bratislava, 46-61.

[444] Patvekar, M.A., Sadana. D. 2014. Pemphigus vulgaris in an elderly patient. *Indian. J. Dermatol.* 59, 105.

[445] Popadic, S., Medenica, L., Skiljevic, D, Djakovic, Z., Nikolic, M. 2011. Pemphigus vulgaris in three adolescents: The course of the disease. *Australas. J. Dermatol.* 52, e3-7.

[446] Hertl, M. 2011. Autoimmune diseases of the skin. Pathogenesis, Diagnosis, Management. Chapter 3. Autoimmunbe bullous skin disorders. 3th Revised Enlarged Edition. Springer Wien NewYork, 33-63.

[447] Shamim, T., Varghese, V.I., Shameena, P.M., Sudha, S. 2008. Pemphigus vulgaris in oral cavity: Clinical analysis of 71 cases. *Med. Oral. Patol. Cir. Bucal.* 13, e622-26.

[448] Scully, C., Mignona, M. 2008. Oral mucosal disease: Pemphigus. *Br. J. Oral. Maxillofac. Surg.* 46, 272-77.

[449] Švecová, D., Danilla, T. 2014. Textbook of dermatology. Chapter 13. Blistering diseases. 2nd Revised Edition. Comenius University, Bratislava, 135-147.

[450] Kneisel, A., Hertl, M. 2011. Autoimmune bullous skin diseases. Part 1. Clinical manifestation. *J. Dtsch. Dermatol. Ges.* 9, 844-57.

[451] Haddayer, N., Ramot, Y., Maly, A., Zlotogorski, A. 2013. Pemphigus vulgaris with loss of hair on the scalp. *Int. J. Trichology* 5, 157-58.

[452] Chmurova, N., Svecova, D. 2009. Pemphigus vulgaris: a 11-year review. *Bratisl. Lek. Listy* 110, 501-504.

[453] Engineer, L., Norton, L.A., Ahmed, A.R. 2000. Nail involvement in pemphigus vulgaris. *J. Am. Acad. Dermatol.* 43, 529-35.

[454] Robati, R.M., Rahmati-Roodsari, M., Dabir-Moghaddam, P., Farnaghi, A., Mahboobi-rad, F., Rahimi, H., Toosi, P. 2012. Mucosal manifestations of pemphigus vulgaris in ear, nose, and throat; before and after treatment. *J. Am. Acad. Dermatol.* 67, e249-52.

[455] España, A., Fernández, S., del Olmo, J., Marquina, M., Pretel, M., Ruba, D., Sánchez-Ibarrola, A. 2007. Ear, nose and throat manifestations in pemphigus vulgaris. *Br. J. Dermatol.* 156, 733-37.

[456] Fernández, S., España, A., Navedo, M., Barona, L. 2012. Study of oral, ear, nose and throat involvement in pemphigus vulgaris by endoscopic examination. *Br. J. Dermatol.* 167, 1011-16.

[457] Kavala, M., Altinas, S., Kocatürk, E., Zindanci, I., Can, B., Ruhi, C., Turkoglu, Z. 2011. Ear, nose and throat involvement in patients with pemphigus vulgaris: correlation with severity, phenotype and disease activity. *J. Eur. Acad. Dermatol. Venereol.* 25, 1324-27.

[458] Mignogna, D.M., Fortuna, G., Leuci, S., Ruoppo, E. 2010. Oropharyngeal pemphigus vulgaris and clinical remission. *Am. J. Clin. Dermatol.* 11, 137-45.

[459] Vasiliou, A., Nikolopoulos, T.P., Manolopoulos, L. 2007. Laryngeal pemphigus without skin manifestation and review of the literature. *Eur. Arch. Otorhinolaryngol.* 264, 509-12.

[460] Mignogna, M.D., Lo Muzio, L., Galloro, G., Satriano, R.A., Ruocco, V., Bucci, E. 1997. Oral pemphigus: clinical significance of esophageal involvement: report of eight cases. *Oral. Surg. Oral. Med. Oral. Pathol. Oral. Radiol. Endod.* 84, 179-84.

[461] Akhyani, M., Keshtkar-Jafari, A., Chams-Davatchi, C., Lajevardi, V., Beigi, S., Aghazadeh, N., Rayati Damavandi, M, Arami, S. 2014. Ocular involvement in pemphigus vulgaris. *J. Dermatol.* 41, 618-21.

[462] Brackley, R., Pagani, J.M. 2011. Conjunctival erosions associated with pemphigus vulgaris. *Optom. Vis. Sci.* 88, 1010-13.

[463] Lifshitz, T., Levy, J., Cagnano, E., Halevy, S. 2004. Severe conjunctival and eyelid involvement in pemphigus vulgaris. *Int. Ophthalmol.* 25, 73-74.

[464] Malik, M., Ahmed, A,R. 2005. Involvement of the female genital tract in pemphigus vulgaris. *Obstet. Gynecol.* 106, 1005-12.

[465] Akhyani, M., Chams-Davatchi, C., Naraghi, Z., Daneshpazhooh, M., Toosi, S., Asgari, M., Malekhami, F. 2008. Cervicovaginal involvement in pemphigus vulgaris: a clinical study of 77 cases. *Br. J. Dermatol.* 158, 478-82.

[466] Sami, N., Ahmed, A.R. 2001. Penile pemphigus. *Arch. Dermatol.* 137, 756-58.

[467] Kherzi, S., Mahmoudi, H.R., Masoom, S.N., Daneshpazhooh, M., Balighi, K., Hosseini, S.H., Chams-Davatchi, S. 2013. Anal involvement in pemphigus vulgaris. *Autoimmune Dis.* 2013, 609181.

[468] Ahmed, A.R., Blose, D.A. 1984. Pemphigus vegetans. Neumann type and Hallopeau type. *Int. J. Dermatol.* 23, 135-41.

[469] Monshi, B., Marker, M., Feichtinger, H., Schmidt, G., Kriehuber, E., Födinger, D., Rappersberger, K. 2010. Pemphigus vegetans-immunopathological findings in a rare variant of pemphigus vulgaris. *J. Dtsch. Dermatol. Ges.* 8, 179-83.

[470] Burgdorf,W. H.C., Plewig, G., Wolf, H.H., Landthaler,M. 2009. Braun-Falco´s Dermatology. Blistering diseases. 3rd Edition. Springer Heidelberg, 625-647.

[471] Daniel, B.S., Hertl, M, Werth, V.P., Eming, R., Murrell, D. 2012. Severity score indexes for blistering diseases. *Clin. Dermatol.* 30, 108-113.

[472] Sabaratnam, D.F., Murrell, D.F. 2011. Objective scoring systems for disease activity in autoimmune bullous disease. *Dermatol. Clin.* 29, 515-520.

[473] Rosenbach, M., Murrell, D.F., Bystryn, J.C., Dulay, S., Dick, S., Fakharzadech, S., Hall, R., Korman, N.J., Lin, J., Okawa, J., Pandya, A.G., Payne, A.S., Rose, M., Rubenstein, D., Woodley, D., Vittorio, C., Werth, B.B., Williams, E.A., Taylor, L., Troxel, A.B., Werth, V.P. 2009. Reliability and convergent validity of two outcome instruments for pemphigus. *J. Invest. Dermatol.* 129, 2404-10.

[474] Bystryn, J.C., Steinman, N.M. 1996. The adjuvant therapy of pemphigus. An update. *Arch. Dermatol.* 132, 203-12.

[475] Bystryn, J.C. 2002. How should pemphigus be treated? *J Eur. Acad. Dermatol. Venereol.* 16, 607-611.

[476] Almugairen, N, Hospital, V., Bedane, C., Duvert-Lehembre, S., Picard, D., Tronquoy, A.F., Houivet, E., D´incan, M., Joly, P.2013. Assessment of the rate of long-term complete remission off therapy in patients with pemphigus treated with different regimens including medium-and high-dose corticosteroids. *J. Am. Acad. Dermatol.* 69, 583-88.

[477] Herbst, A, Bystryn, J.C. 2000. Patterns of remission in pemphigus vulgaris. *J. Am. Acad. Dermatol.* 42, 422-27.

[478] Murrell, D.F., Dick, S., Ahmed, A.R., Amagai, M., Barnadas, M.A., Borradori, L., Bystryn, J.C., Cianchini, G., Diaz, L., Fivenson, D., Hall, R., Harman, K.E., Hashimoto, T., Hertl, M., Hunzelmann, N., Iranzo, P., Joly, P., Jonkman, M.F., Kitajima, Y., Korman, N.J., Martin, L.K., Mimouni, D., Sinha, A.A., Sirois, D., Zillikens, D., Werth, V.P. 2008. Consensus statement on definitions of disease, end points, and therapeutic response for pemphigus. *J. Am. Acad. Dermatol.* 58, 1043-46.

[479] Ioannides, D., Chrysomallis, F., Bystryn, J.C. 2000. Ineffectiveness of cyclosporine as an adjuvant to corticosteroids in the treatment of pemphigus. *Arch. Dermatol.* 136, 868-72.

[480] Nguyen, V.T., Arredondo, J., Chernyavsky, A.I., Kitajima, Y., Pittelkow, M. Grando, S.A. 2004. Pemphigus vulgaris IgG and methylprednisolone exhibit reciprocal effects on keratinocytes. *J. Biol. Chem.* 16, 279, 2135-46.

[481] Hertl, M., Jedlickova, H., Karpati, S, Marinovic, B., Uzun, S., Yali, S., Mimouni, D., Borradori, L., Feliciani, C., Ioannides, D., Joly, P., Kowalewski, C., Zambruno, G., Zillikens, D., Jonkman, M.F. 2014. Pemphigus. S2 Guideline for diagnosis and treatment -guided by the European Dermatology Forum (EDF) in cooperation with the European Academy of Dermatology and Venereology (EADV). *J. Eur. Acad. Dermatol. Venereol.* doi 10.1111/jdv.12772.

[482] Harman, K.E., Albert, S., Black, M.M. 2003. Guidelines for the management of pemphigus vulgaris. *Br. J. Dermatol.* 149, 926-37.

[483] Ratnam, K.V., Phay, K.L., Tan, C.K. 1990. Pemphigus therapy with oral prednisolone regimens. A 5-years study. *Int. J. Dermatol.* 29, 363-67.

[484] Lever, W., White, H. 1963. Treatment of pemphigus with corticosteroids results obtained in 46 patients over a period of 11 years. *Arch. Dermatol.* 87, 12-26.

[485] Werth, V.P. 1996. Treatment of pemphigus vulgaris with brief, high-dose intravenous glucocorticoids. *Arch. Dermatol.* 132, 1435-39.

[486] Roujeau, J.C. 1996. Pulse glucorticoid therapy. The ´big shot´ revisited. *Arch. Dermatol.* 132, 1499-502.

[487] Mutasin, D.F. 2004. Management of autoimmune bullous diseases: Pharmacology and therapeutics. *J. Am. Acad. Dermatol.* 51, 859-77.

[488] Truhan, A.P., Ahmed, A.R. 1989. Corticosteroids: a review with emphasis on complications of prolonged systemic therapy. *Ann. Allergy.* 62, 375-91.

[489] Chrysomallis, F., Ioannides, D., Teknetzis, A., Panagiotidou, D., Minas, A. 1994. Treatment of oral pemphigus vulgaris. *Int. J. Derma*tol. 33, 803-7.

[490] Chaidemenos, G., Apalla, Z., Koussidou, T., Papagarifallou, I., Ioannides. D. 2011. High dose oral prednisone vs. prednisone plus azathioprine for the treatment of oral pemphigus: a retrospective, bi-centre, comparative study. *J. Eur. Acad. Dermatol. Venereol.* 25, 206-10.

[491] Chams-Davatchi, C., Mortazavizadeh, A., Daneshpazhooh, M., Davatchi, F., Balighi, K., Esmaili, N., Akhyani, M., Hallaji, Z., Seirafi, H., Mortazavi, H. 2013. Randomized double blind trial of prednisolone and azathioprine, vs. prednisolone and placebo, in the treatment of pemphigus vulgaris *J. Eur. Acad. Dermatol. Venereol.* 27, 1285-92.

[492] Chams-Davatchi, C, Esmaili, N., Daneshpazhooh, M., Valikhani, M., Balighi, K., Hallaji, Z., Barzegari, M., Akhyani, M., Ghodsi, S.Z., Seifari, H., Nazemi, M.J., Mortazavi, H., Mirshams-Shahshahani, M. 2007. Randomized controlled open-label trial of four treatment regimens for pemphigus vulgaris. *J. Am. Acad. Dermatol.* 57, 622-28.

[493] Schiavo, A.L., Puca, R.V., Ruocco, V., Ruocco, E. 2010. Adjuvant drugs in autoimmune bullous diseases, efficacy versus safety: Facts and controversies. *Clin. Dermatol.* 28, 337-43.

[494] Patel, A.A., Swerlick, R.A., McCall, C.O. 2006. Azathioprine in dermatology: the past, the present, and future. *J. Am. Acad. Dermatol.* 55, 369-89.

[495] Anstey, A.V., Wakelin, S., Reynolds, N.J. 2004. Guidelines for prescribing azathioprine in dermatology. *Br. J. Dermatol.* 151, 1123-32.

[496] Mauer, M. 2012. Immunosuppressive therapy for autoimmune bullous disease. *Clin. Dermatol.* 30, 78-83.

[497] Tichy, M., Urbanek, J., Sternbersky, J., Ditrichova, D., Hercogova, J. 2014. Life-threatening course of pemphigus vulgaris complicated by sepsis caused by azathioprine-induced bone marrow suppression, successfully managed with combination therapy. *Dermatol. Ther.* 27, 183-86.

[498] Orvis, A.K, Wesson, S.K., Breza, T.S., Church, A.A., Mitchell, C.L., Watkins, S.W. 2009. Mycophenolate mofetil in dermatology. *J. Am. Acad. Dermatol.* 60, 183-99.

[499] Enk, A.H., Knop. J. 1999. Mycophenolate is effective in the treatment of pemphigus vulgaris. *Arch. Dermatol.* 135, 54-56.

[500] Beissert, S., Werfel, T., Frieling, U., Böhm, M., Sticherling, M., Stadler, R., Zillinkens, D., Rzany, B., Hunzelmann, N., Meurer, M., Gollnick, H., Ruzicka, T., Pillekamp, H., Junghans, V., Luger, T.A. 2006. A comparison of oral methylprednisolone plus azathioprine or mycophenolate mofetil for the treatment of pemphigus. *Arch. Dermatol.* 142, 1447-54.

[501] Ishikawa, H. 1999. Mizoribine and mycophenolate mofetil. *Curr. Med. Chem.* 6, 575-97.

[502] Yokota, S. 2002. Mizoribine: Mode of action and effects in clinical use. *Pediatr. Int.* 44, 196-98.

[503] Hashimoto, T., Kawakami, T., Koga, H., Ohyama, B., Hamada, T., Dainichi, T., Nakama, T., Yasumoto, S., Tsuruta, D., Ishii. N. 2012. Therapeutic effect of mizoribine on pemphigus vulgaris and pemphigus foliaceus. *Dermatol. Ther.* 25, 382-85.

[504] Pasricha, J.S., Sood, V.D., Minocha, Y. 1975. Treatment of pemphigus with cyclophosphamide. *Br. J. Dermatol.* 93, 573-76.

[505] Ahmed, A.R, Hombal, S. 1987. Use of cyclophosphamide in azathioprine failures in pemphigus. *J. Am. Acad. Derm*atol. 17, 437-42.

[506] Fellner, M.J., Katz, J.M., McCabe, J.B. 1978. Successful use of cyclophosphamide and prednisone for initial treatment of pemphigus vulgaris. *Arch. Dermatol.* 114, 889-94.

[507] Pasricha, J.S., Das, S.S. 1992. Curative effect of dexamethasone-cyclophosphamide pulse therapy for the treatment of pemphigus vulgaris. *Int. J. Dermatol.* 31, 875-77.

[508] Pasricha, J.S., Thanzama, J., Khan, U.K. 1988. Intermittent high-dose dexamethasone-cyclophosphamide therapy for pemphigus. *Br. J. Dermatol.* 119, 73-77.

[509] Olszewska, M., Kolacinska-Strasz, Z., Sulej, J., Labecka, H., Cwikla, J., Natorska, U., Blaszczyk, M. 2007. Efficacy and safety of cyclophosphamide, azathioprine, and cyclosporine (ciclosporin) as adjuvant drugs in pemphigus vulgaris. *Am. J. Clin. Dermatol.* 8, 85-92.

[510] Gürcan, H.M., Ahmed, A.R. 2009. Analysis of current data on the use of methotrexate in the treatment of pemphigus and pemphigoid. *Br. J. Dermatol.* 161, 723-31.

[511] Lever, W.F. 1972. Methotrexate and prednisone in pemphigus vulgaris therapeutic results obtained in 36 patients between 1961 and 1970. *Arch. Dermatol.* 106, 491-97.

[512] Bangert, C.A., Costner, M.I. 2007. Methotrexate in dermatology. *Dermatol. Ther.* 20, 216-228.

[513] Tran, K.D., Wolverton, J.E. Soter, N.A. 2013. Methotrexate in the treatment of pemphigus vulgaris: experience in 23 patients. *Br. J. Dermatol.* 169, 916-21.

[514] Mashkilleyson, N., Mashkilleyson, A.L. 1988. Mucous membrane manifestations of pemphigus vulgaris. A 25-year survey of 185 patients treated with corticosteroids or with combination of corticosteroids with methotrexate or heparin. *Acta Derm. Venereol.* 68, 413-21.

[515] Smith, T.J., Bystryn, J.C. 1999. Methotrexate as an adjuvant treatment for pemphigus vulgaris. *Arch. Dermatol.* 135, 1275-76.

[516] Kuitunen, T., Malmström, J., Palva, E., Pettersson, T. 2005. Pancytopenia induced by low-dose methotrexate. A study of the cases reported to the Finish Adverse Drug Reaction Register from 1991to 1999. *Scand. J. Rheumatol.* 34, 238-41.

[517] Liddle, B.J. 1991. Methotrexate interactions. *Clin. Exp. Dermatol.* 16, 311-12.

[518] El-Sheikh, A.A., van de Heuvel, J.J., Koenderink, J.B., Russel, F.G. 2007. Interaction of nonsteroidal anti-inflammatory drugs with multidrug resistance protein (MRP) 2/ABCC2-and MRP4/ABCC4-mediated methotrexate transport. *J. Pharmacol. Exp. Ther.* 320, 229-35.

[519] Van Dooren-Greebe, R.J., Kuijpers, A.L., Mulder, J., De Boo, T., Van de Kerkhof, P.C. 1994. Methotrexate revisited: effects of long-term treatment in psoriasis. *Br. J. Dermatol.* 130, 204-10.

[520] Shen, S., O´Brien, T., Yap, L.M., Prince, H.M., McCormack, C.J. 2012. The use of methotrexate in dermatology: a review. *Australas. J. Dermatol.* 55, 1-18.

[521] Chalmers, R.J., Kirby, B., Smith, A., Burrows, P., Little, R., Horan, M., Hextall, J.M., Smith, C.H., Klaber, M., Rogers, S. 2005. Replacement of routine liver biopsy by procollagen III amonipeptide for monitoring patients with psoriasis receiving long-term methotrexate: a multicentre audit and health economic analysis. *Br. J. Dermatol.* 152, 444-50.

[522] Kalb, R.E., Strober, B., Weinstein, G., Lebwohl, M. 2009. Methotrexate and psoriasis: 2009 National Psoriasis Foundation Consensus Conference. *J. Am. Acad. Dermatol.* 60, 824-37.

[523] Donnenfeld, A.E., Pastuszak, A., Noah, J.S., Schick, B., Rose, N.C., Koren, G. 1994. Methotrexate exposure prior to and during pregnancy. *Teratology* 49, 79-81.

[524] Gwak, G.Y., Koh, K.C., Kim, H.Y. 2007. Fatal hepatic failure associated with hepatitis B virus reactivation in a hepatitis B surface antigen-negative patients with rheumatoid arthritis receiving low dose methotrexate. *Clin. Exp. Rheumatol.* 25, 888-89.

[525] Binymin, K,, Cooper, R.G. 2001. Late reactivation of spinal tuberculosis by low-dose methotrexate therapy in a patient with rheumatoid arthritis. *Rheumatology* 40, 341-42.

[526] Kalantzis, A., Marschman, Z., Falconer, D.T., Morgan, P.R., Odell, E.W. 2005. Oral effects of low-dose methotrexate treatment. *Oral. Surg. Oral. Med. Oral. Pathol. Oral. Radiol. Endod.* 100, 52-62.

[527] Kazlow, D.W., Federgrun, D., Kurtin, S., Lebwohl, M.G. 2003. Cutaneous ulceration caused by methotrexate. *J. Am. Acad. Dermatol.* 49, S197-98.

[528] Barthelemy, H., Frappaz, A., Cambazard, F., Mauduit, G., Rouchouse, B., Kanitakis, J., Souteyrand, P., Claudy, A.L.,Thivolet, J. 1988. Treatment of nine cases of pemphigus vulgaris with cyclosporine. *J. Am. Acad. Dermatol.* 18, 1262-66.

[529] Alijotas, J., Pedragosa, R., Bosch, J., Vilardell, M. 1990. Prolonged remission after cyclosporine therapy in pemphigus vulgaris: report of two young siblings. *J. Am. Acad. Dermatol.* 23, 701-3.

[530] Lapidoth, M., David, M., Ben-Amitai, D., Katzenelson, V., Lustig, S., Sandbank, M.1994. The efficacy of combined treatment with prednisone and cyclosporine in patients with pemphigus: preliminary study. *J. Am. Acad. Dermatol.* 30, 752-57.

[531] Hubert, P., Treffel, P., Chapuis, J.F., Buchet, S., Derancourt, C., Agache, P. 1991. The tetracycline in dermatology. *J. Am. Acad. Dermatol.* 25, 691-97.

[532] Ungerstedt, J.S., Blombäck, M., Söderström, T. 2003. Nicotinamide is a potent inhibitor of proinflammatory cytokines. *Clin. Exp. Immunol.* 131, 48-52.

[533] Hornschuh, B., Hamm, H., Wever, S., Hashimoto, T., Schöder, U., Bröcker, E.B., Zillikens, D. 1997. Treatment of 16 patients with bullous pemphigoid with oral tetracycline and niacinamide and topical clobetasol. *J. Am. Acad. Dermatol.* 36, 101-3.

[534] Chaffins, M.L., Collison, D., Fivenson, D.P. 1993. Treatment of pemphigus and linear IgA dermatosis with nicotinamide and tetracycline: a review of 13 cases. *J. Am. Acad. Dermatol.* 23, 998-1000.

[535] McCarty, M., Fivenson, D., Arbor, A. 2014. Two decades of using the combination of tetracycline derivates and niacinamide as steroid-sparing agents in the management of pemphigus: defining a niche for these toxicity agents. *J. Am. Acad. Dermatol.* 71, 475-79.

[536] Calebotta, A., Sáenz, A.M., González, F., Carvalho, M., Castillo, R. 1999. Pemphigus vulgaris: benefits of tetracycline as adjuvant therapy in a series of thirteen patients. *Int. J. Dermatol.* 38, 217-21.

[537] Wozel, G., Blasum, C. 2014. Dapsone in dermatology and beyond. *Arch. Dermatol.* 306, 103-24.

[538] Chen, X.Y., Buschmann, H., Bolm, C. 2012. Sulfoximine - and Sulfilimine- based Dapson analogues; syntheses and bioactivities. *SYNLETT* 23, 2808-10.

[539] Piamphongsant, T. 1976. Pemphigus controlled by dapsone. *Br. J. Dermatol.* 94, 681-86.

[540] Hain, S., Friedman-Birnbaum, R. 1978. Dapsone in the treatment of pemphigus vulgaris. *Dermatologica* 156, 120-23.

[541] Thomas, I. 1987. Gold therapy and its indications in dermatology. A review. *J. Am. Acad. Dermatol.* 16, 845-54.

[542] Pandya, A.G., Dyke, C. 1998. Treatment of pemphigus with gold. *Arch. Dermatol.* 134, 1104-7.

[543] Iranzo, P., Alsina, M.M., Martinez-De Pablo, I., Segura, S., Mascaró, J.M., Herrero, C. 2007. Gold: an old drug till working in refractory pemphigus. *J. Eur. Acad. Dermatol.* 21, 902-7.

[544] Lange, D., Meiss, F., Fiedler, F., Fiedler, E., Marsch, W.C., Fischer, M. 2007. Gold Effektive Therapie bei Schleimhautläsionen des Pemphigus vulgaris. *Hautarzt* 58, 142-45.

[545] Roujeau, J.C. 1988. Plasmapheresis therapy of pemphigus and bullous pemphigoid. *Semin. Dermatol.* 7, 195-200.

[546] Perez, O.A., Patton, T. 2009. Novel therapies for pemphigus vulgaris. *Drugs Aging* 26, 833-46.

[547] Meurer, M., Messer, G. 2002. Plasmapheresis and intravenous immunoglobulin. *Dermatol. Ther.* 15, 333-39.

[548] Turner, M.S., Sutton, D., Sauder, D.N. 2000. The use of plasmapheresis and immunosuppresion in the treatment of pemphigus vulgaris. *J. Am. Acad. Dermatol.*43, 1058-64.

[549] Sondergaard, K., Carstens, J., Jorgensen, J., Zachariae, H. 1995. The steroid-sparing effect of long-term plasmapheresis in pemphigus. *Acta Derm. Venereol.* 75, 150-2.

[550] Sagi, L., Baum, S., Gendelman, V., Trau, H., Barzilai, A. 2011. The role of therapeutic plasma exchange in pemphigus vulgaris. *J. Eur. Acad. Dermatol. Venereol.* 25, 82-86.

[551] Guillaume, J.C., Roujeau, J.C., Morel, P., Doutre, M.S., Guillot, B., Lambert, D., Lauret, P., Lorette, G., Prigent, F., Triller, T. 1988. Controlled study of plasma exchange in pemphigus. *Arch. Dermatol.* 124, 1659-63.

[552] Braun, N., Bosch, T. 2000. Immunoadsorption, current status and future development. *Expert. Opin. Investig. Drugs.* 9, 2017-38.

[553] Amagai, M, Hashimoto, T., Shimizu, N., Nishikawa, T. 1994. Absorption of pathogenic autoantibodies by the extracellular domain of pemphigus vulgaris antigen (Dsg3) produced by baculovirus. *J. Clin. Invest.* 94, 59-67.

[554] Schmidt, E., Zillikens, D. 2010. Immunoadsorption in dermatology. *Arch. Dermatol. Res.* 302, 241-53.

[555] Eming, R., Rech, J., Barth, S., Kalden, J.R., Schuler, G., Harrer, T., Hertl, M. 2006. Prolonged clinical remission of patients with severe pemphigus upon rapid removal of desmoglein-reactive autoantibodies by immunoadsorption. *Dermatology* 212, 177-87.

[556] Lüftl, M., Stauber, A., Mainka, A., Klingel, R., Schuller, G., Hertl, M. 2003. Successful removal of pathogenic autoantibodies in pemphigus by immunoadsorption with tryptophan-linked polyvinylalcohol adsorber. *Br. J. Dermatol.* 149, 598-605.

[557] Schmidt, E., Klinker, E., Opitz, A., Herzog, S., Sitaru, C., Goebeler, M., Mansouri Taleghoni, B., Bröcker, E.B., Zillikens, D. 2003. Protein A immunoadsorption: a novel and effective adjuvant treatment of severe pemphigus. *Br. J. Dermatol.* 148, 1222-29.

[558] Shimanovich, I., Herzog, S., Schmidt, E., Opitz, A., Klinker, E., Bröcker, E.B., Goebeler, M., Zillikens. D. 2006. Improved protocol for treatment of pemphigus vulgaris with protein A immunoadsorption. *Clin. Exp. Dermatol.* 31, 768-74.

[559] Meyersburg, D., Schmidt, E., Kasperkiewicz, M., Zillikens, D. 2012. Immunoadsorption in dermatology. *Ther. Apher. Dial.* 16, 311-20.

[560] Clynes, R. 2007. Protective mechanisms of IVIG. *Curr. Opin. Immunol.* 19, 646-51.

[561] Smith, S.D., Dennington, P.M., Cooper, A. 2010. The use of intravenous immunoglobulin for treatment of dermatological conditions in Australia: a review. *Australas. J. Dermatol.* 51, 227-37.

[562] Chee, S.N., Murrell, D.F. 2011. The use of intravenous immunoglobulin in autoimmune bullous diseases. *Dermatol. Clin.* 29, 565-70.

[563] Enk, A., European Dermatology Forum Guideline Subcommittee. 2009. Guidelines of the use of high-dose intravenous immunoglobulin in dermatology. *Eur. J. Dermatol.* 19, 90-98.

[564] Sibéril, S., Elluru, S., Negi, V.S., Ephrem, A., Misra, N., Delignat, S., Bayary, J., Lacroix-Desmazes, S., Kazatchikine, M.D., Kaveri, S.V. 2007. Intravenous immunoglobulin in autoimmune and inflammatory diseases: More than mere transfer of antibodies. *Transfus. Apher.* Sci. 37, 103-107.

[565] Mimouni, D., Blank, M., Payne, A.S., Anhalt, G.J., Avivi, C., Barshack, I., David, M., Shoenfeld, Y. 2010. Efficacy of intravenous immunoglobulin (IVIG) affinity-purified anti-desmoglein anti-idiotypic antibodies in the treatment of an experimental model of pemphigus vulgaris. *Clin. Exp. Immunol.* 162, 543-49.

[566] Mimouni, D., Blank, M., Ashkenazi, L., Milner, Y., Frusic-Zlotkin, M., Anhalt, G.J., David, M., Shoenfeld, Y. 2005. Protective effect of intravenous immunoglobulin (IVIG) in an experimental model of pemphigus vulgaris. *Clin. Exp. Immunol.* 142, 426-32.

[567] Kimberly, R.P., Salmon, J.E., Bussel, J.B., Crow, M.K., Hilgartner, M.W. 1984. Modulation on mononuclear phagocyte function by intravenous gammaglobulin. *J. Immunol.* 132, 745-50.

[568] van Mirre, E., Teeling, J.L., van der Meer, J.W., Blecker, W.K., Hack, C.E. 2004. Monomeric IgG in intravenous Ig preparations is a functional antagonist of FcγRII and FcγRIIIb. *J. Immunol.* 173, 332-39.

[569] Boruchov, A.M., Heller, G., Veri, M.C., Bonvini, E., Ravetch, J.V., Young, J.W. 2005. Activation and inhibitory IgG Fc receptors on human DCs mediate opposing functions. *J. Clin. Invest.* 115, 2914-23.

[570] Aoyama, Y. 2010. What´s new in i.v. immunoglobulin therapy and pemphigus: High-dose i.v. immunoglobulin therapy and its mode of action for treatment of pemphigus. *J. Dermatol.* 37, 239-45.

[571] Akilesh, S., Petkova, S., Sproule, T.J., Shaffer, D.J., Christianson, G.J., Roopenian, D. 2004. The MHC class I-like Fc receptor promotes humorally mediated autoimmune disease. *J. Clin. Invest.* 113, 1328-33.

[572] de Souza, R., Carreno, M.P., Kaveri, S.V., Ledur, A., Sadeghi, H., Cavaillon, J.M., Kzatchkine, M.D., Haeffner-Cavaillon, N. 1995. Selective induction of interleukin-1 antagonist and interleukin-8 in human monocytes by normal polyspecific IgG (intravenous immunoglobulin). *Eur. J. Immunol.* 25, 1267-73.

[573] Toosi, S., Habib, N, Torres, G., Reynolds, S.R., Bystryn, J.C. 2011. Serum levels of inhibitors of apoptotic proteins (IAPs) change with IVIg therapy in pemphigus. *J. Invest. Dermatol.* 131, 2327-29.

[574] Viard, I., Wehrli, P., Bullani, R., Scheider, P., Holler, N., Salomon, D., Hunziker, T., Saurat, J.H., Tschopp, J., French, L.E. 1998. Inhibition of toxic epidermal necrolysis by blockade of CD95 with human intravenous immunoglobulin. *Science* 282, 490-93.

[575] Bayry, J., Lacroix-Desmazes, S., Carbonneil, C., Misra, N., Donkova, V., Pashov, A., Chevailler, A., Mouthon, L., Weill, B., Bruneval, P., Kazatchkine, M.D., Kaveri, S.V. 2003. Inhibition of maturation and function of dendritic cells by intravenous immunoglobulin. *Blood* 101, 758-65.

[576] Czernik, A., Toosi, S., Bystryn, J.C., Grando, S.A. 2012. Intravenous immunoglobulin in the treatment of autoimmune bullous dermatoses: an update. *Autoimmunity* 45, 111-18.

[577] Kasperkiewicz, M., Schmidt, E., Zillikens, D. 2012. Current therapy of the pemphigus group. *Clin. Dermatol.* 30, 84-94.

[578] Green, G.M., Bystryn, J.C. 2008. Effect of intravenous immunoglobulin therapy on serum levels of IgG1 and IgG4 antidesmoglein 1 and antidesmoglein 3 antibodies in pemphigus vulgaris. *Arch. Dermatol.* 144, 1621-24.

[579] Amagai, M., Ikeda, S., Shimizu, H., Pemphigus Study Group Japan. 2009. A randomized double-blind trial of intravenous immunoglobulin for pemphigus. *J. Am. Acad. Dermatol.* 60, 595-603.

[580] Gürcan, H.M., Jeph, S., Ahmed, R. 2010. Intravenous immunoglobulin therapy in autoimmune mucocutaneous blistering diseases. *Am. J. Clin. Dermatol.* 11, 315-26.

[581] Sami, N., Qureshi, A., Ruocco, E., Ahmed, A.R. 2002. Corticosteroid-sparing effect on intravenous immunoglobulin therapy in patients with pemphigus vulgaris. *Arch. Dermatol.* 138, 1158-62.

[582] Baum, S., Scope, A., Barzilai, A., Azizi, E., Trau, H. 2006. The role of IVIg treatment in severe pemphigus vulgaris. *J. Eur. Acad. Dermatol. Venereol.* 20, 548-52.

[583] Švecová, D. 2014. Intravenous immunoglobulin (IVIG) therapy in pemphigus. (Liečba pemfigu intravenóznymi imunoglobulínmi (IVIG). *Ces Dermatovenerol.* 4, 221-223.

[584] Lolis, M., Toosi, S., Czernik, A., Bystryn, J.C. 2011. Effect of intravenous immunoglobulin with or without cytotoxic drugs on pemphigus intercellular antibodies. *J. Am. Acad. Dermatol.* 64, 484-89.

[585] Ahmed, A.R., Gürcan, H.M. 2011. Use of intravenous immunoglobulin therapy during pregnancy in patients with pemphigus vulgaris. *J. Eur. Acad. Dermatol. Venereol.* 25, 1073-79.

[586] Asarch, A., Ahmed, A.R. 2009. Treatment of juvenile pemphigus vulgaris with intravenous immunoglobulin therapy. *Pediatr. Dermatol.* 26, 197-202.

[587] Seidling, V., Hoffmann, J.H., Enk, A.H., Hadaschik, E.N. 2013. Analysis of high-dose intravenous immunoglobulin therapy in 16 patients with refractory autoimmune blistering skin disease: high efficacy and no serious adverse events. *Acta Derm. Venereol.* 93, 346-49.

[588] Stiehm, E.R. 2013. Adverse effects of human immunoglobulin therapy. *Transfus. Med. Rev.* 27, 171-78.

[589] Rachid, R., Bonilla, F.A. 2012. The role of anti-IgA antibodies in causing adverse reactions to gamma globulin infusion in immunodeficient patients: A comparative review of the literature. *J. Allergy Clin. Immunol.* 129, 628-34.

[590] Scriber, C.L., Kapit, R.M., Phillips, E.T., Rickles, N.M. 1994. Aseptic meningitis and intravenous immunoglobulin therapy. *Ann. Intern. Med.* 121, 305-306.

[591] Mignogna, M.D., Fortuna, G., Leuci, S., Ruoppo, E., Adamo, D., Fedele, S. 2008. Analysis of thromboembolic risk related to high-dose intravenous immunoglobulin treatment: a preliminary clinical study of 10 patients with autoimmune mucocutaneous blistering diseases. *Clin. Exp. Dermatol.* 34, 145-50.

[592] Borradori, L., Lombardi, T., Samson, J., Girardet, C., Saurat, J.H., Hügli, A. 2001. Anti-CD20 monoclonal antibody (rituximab) for refractory erosive stomatitis secondary to CD20 (+) follicular lymphoma-associated paraneoplastic pemphigus. *Arch. Dermatol.* 137, 269-72.

[593] Taylor, R.P., Lindorfer, M.A. 2007. Drug insight: the mechanism of action of rituximab in autoimmune disease-the immune complex decoy hypothesis. *Nat. Clin. Pract. Rheumatol.* 3, 86-95.

[594] Golay, J., Zaffaroni, L., Vaccari, T., Lazzari, M., Borleri, G.M., Bernasconi, S., Tedesco, F., Rambaldi, A., Introna, M. 2000. Biologic response of B lymphoma cells to anti-CD20 monoclonal antibody rituximab in vitro: CD55 and CD29 regulate complement-mediated cell lysis. *Blood* 95, 3900-3908.

[595] Lefebvre, M.L., Krause, S.W., Salcedo, M., Nardin, A. 2006. Ex vivo-activated human macrophages kill chronic lymphocytic leukemia cells in the presence of rituximab: mechanism of antibody-dependent cellular cytotoxicity and impact of human serum. *J. Immunonother.* 29, 388-97.

[596] Gürcan, H.M., Keskin, D.B., Stern, J.N., Nitzberg, M.A., Shekhani, H., Ahmed, A.R. 2008. A review of the current use of rituximab in autoimmune diseases. *Int. Immunopharmacol.* 9, 10-25.

[597] Sfikakis, P.P., Souliotis, V.L., Fragiadaki, K.G., Moutsopoulos, H.M., Boletis, J.N., Theofilopoulos, A.N. 2007. Increased expression of the FoxP3 functional marker of regulatory T cells following B cell depletion with rituximab in patients with lupus nephritis. *Clin. Immunol.* 123, 66-77.

[598] Raimondi, G., Zanoni, I., Citterio, S., Ricciardi-Castagnoli, P., Granucci, F. 2006. Induction of peripheral T cell tolerance by antigen-presenting B cells. II. Chronic antigen presentation overrules antigen-presenting B cell activation. *J. Immunol.* 176, 4021-28.

[599] Arin, M.J., Engert, A., Krieg, T., Hunzelmann, N. 2005. Anti-CD20 monoclonal antibody (rituximab) in the treatment of pemphigus. *Br. J. Dermatol.* 153, 620-25.

[600] Bai, S., Jorga, K., Xin, Y., Jin, D., Zheng, Y., Damico-Beyer, L.A., Gupta, M., Tang, M., Allison, D.E., Lu, D., Zhang, Y., Joshi, A., Dresser, M.J. 2012. A guide to rational dosing of monoclonal antibodies. *Clin. Pharmacokinet.* 51, 119-35.

[601] Hertl, M., Zillikens, D., Borradori, L., Brucker-Tuderman, L., Burckhard, H., Eming, R., Engert, A., Goebeler, M., Hofmann, S., Hunzelmann, N., Karlhofer, F., Kautz, O., Niedermeier, A., Nitschke, M., Pfütze, M., Reiser, M., Rose, C., Schmidt, E., Shimanovich, I., Sticherling, M., Wolff-Franke, S. 2008. Recommendations for the use of rituximab (anti-CD20 antibody) in the treatment of autoimmune bullous skin diseases. *J. Dtsch. Dermatol. Ges.* 6, 366-73.

[602] Joly, P., Mouquet, H., Roujeau, J.C., D´Incan, M., Gilbert, D., Jacquot, S., Gougeon, M.L., Bedane, C., Muller, R., Dreno, B., Doutre, M.S., Delaporte, E., Pauweis, C., Franck, N., Caux, F., Picard, C., Tancrede-Bohin, E., Bernard, P., Tron, F., Hertl, M., Musette, P. 2007. A single cycle of rituximab for the treatment of severe pemphigus. *N. Engl. J. Med.* 357, 545-52.

[603] Ahmed, A.R., Spigelman, Z., Cavacini, L.A., Posner, M.R. 2006. Treatment of pemphigus vulgaris with rituximab and intravenous immune globulin. *N. Engl. J. Med.* 355, 1772-79.

[604] Lunardon, L., Tsai, K.J., Propert, K.J., Fett, N., Stanley, J.R., Werth, V.P., Tsai, D.E., Payne, A.S. 2012. Adjuvant rituximab therapy of pemphigus: a single center experience with 31 patients. *Arch. Dermatol.* 148, 1031-36.

[605] Reguiai, Z., Tabary, T., Maizieres, M., Bernard, P. 2012. Rituximab treatment of severe pemphigus: long-term results including immunologic follow-up. *J. Am. Acad. Dermatol.* 67, 623-29.

[606] Leshem, Y.A., Hodak, E., David, M., Anhalt, G.J., Mimouni, D. 2013. Successful treatment of pemphigus with biweekly 1-g infusions of rituximab: a retrospective study of 47 patients. *J. Am. Acad. Dermatol.* 68, 404-11.

[607] Horváth, B., Huizinga, J., Pas, H.H., Mulder, A.B., Jonkman, M.F. 2012. Low-dose rituximab is effective in pemphigus. *Br. J. Dermatol.* 166, 405-12.

[608] Matsukura, S., Knowles, S.R., Walsh, S., Shear, N.H. 2012. Effect of a single-cycle alternative dosing regimen for rituximab for recalcitrant pemphigus. *Arch. Dermatol.* 148, 734 -39.

[609] Kanwar, A.J., Vinay, K., Sawatkar, G.U., Dogra, S., Minz, R.W., Shear, N.H., Koga, H., Ishii, N., Hashimoto, T. 2014. Clinical and immunological outcomes of high- and low dose rituximab treatments in patients with pemphigus: a randomized, comparative, observer-blinded study. *Br. J. Dermatol.* 170, 341-49.

[610] Fledman, R.J., Christen, W.G., Ahmed, A.R. 2012. Comparison of immunological parameters in patients with pemphigus vulgaris following rituximab and IVIG therapy. *Br. J. Dermatol.* 166, 511-17.

[611] Shimanovich, I., Nitschke, M., Rose, C., Grabbe, J., Zillikens, D. 2008. Treatment of severe pemphigus with protein A immunoadsorption, rituximab and intravenous immunoglobulins. *Br. J. Dermatol.* 158, 382-88.

[612] Kimby, E. 2005. Tolerability and safety of rituximab (MabThera®). *Cancer Treat. Rev.* 31, 456-73.

[613] Lemieux, B., Bouafia, F., Thieblemont, C., Hequet, O., Arnaud, P., Tartas, S., Traulle, C., Salles, G., Coiffier, B. 2004. Second treatment with rituximab in B-cell non-

Hodgkin´s lymphoma: efficacy and toxicity on 41 patients treated at CHU-Lyon Sud. *Hematol.* J.5, 467-71.

[614] Seror, R., Sordet, C., Guillevin, L., Hachulla, E., Masson, C., Ittah, M., Condon, S., Le Guern, V., Aouba, A., Sibilia, J., Gottenberg, J.E., Mariette, X. 2007. Tolerance and efficacy of rituximab and changes in serum B cell biomarkers in patients with systemic complications of primary Sjögren´s syndrome. *Ann. Rheum. Dis.* 66, 351-57.

[615] Westerhof, W. 1989. Treatment of bullous pemphigoid with topical clobetasol propionate. *J. Am. Acad. Dermatol.* 20, 458-61.

[616] Gutfreund, K., Bienias, W., Szewczyk, A., Kaszuba, A. 2013. Topical calcineurin inhibitors in dermatology. Part I: properties, method and effectiveness of drug use. *Postepy Dermatol. Alergol.* 30, 165-69.

[617] Hodgson, T.A., Malik, F., Hegarty, A.M., Porter, S.R. 2003. Topical tacrolimus: a novel therapeutic intervention for recalcitrant labial pemphigus vulgaris. *Eur. J. Dermatol.* 13, 142-44.

[618] Termeer, C.C., Technau, K., Augustin, M., Simon, J.C. 2004. Topical tacrolimus (protopic) for the treatment of a localized pemphigus foliaceus. *J. Eur. Acad. Dermatol. Venereol.* 18, 636-45.

[619] Gach, J.E., Ilchyshyn, A. 2004. Beneficial effects of topical tacrolimus on recalcitrant erosions of pemphigus vulgaris. *Clin. Exp. Dermatol.* 29, 271-72.

[620] Tyros, G., Kalapothakou, K., Christofidou, E., Kanelleas, A., Stavropoulos, P.G. 2013. Successful treatment of localized pemphigus foliaceus with topical pimecrolimus. *Case Rep. Dermatol. Med.* 2013, 489618.

[621] Iraji, F., Asilian, A., Siadat, A.H. 2010. Pimercolimus 1% cream in the treatment of cutaneous lesions of pemphigus vulgaris: a double-blind, placebo-controlled clinical trial. *J. Drugs. Dermatol.* 9, 684-86.

[622] Tsang, M.W., Wong, W.K., Hung, C.S., Lai, K.M., Tang, W., Cheung, E.Y., Kam, G., Leung, L., Chan, C.W., Chu, C.M., Lam, E.K. 2003. Human epidermal growth factor enhances healing of diabetic foot ulcers. *Diabetes Care* 26, 1856-61.

[623] Fu, X., Li, X., Cheng, B., Chen, W., Sheng, Z. 2005. Engineered growth factors and cutaneous wound healing: success and possible questions in the past 10 years. *Wound Repair. Regen.* 13, 122-30.

[624] Tabrizi, M.N., Chams-Davatchi, C., Esmaeeli, N., Noormohammadpoor, P., Safar, F., Etemadzadeh, H. 2006. Accelerating effects of epidermal growth factor on skin lesions of pemphigus vulgaris: a double-blind, randomized, controlled trial. *J. Eur. Acad. Dermatol. Venereol.* 21, 79-84.

[625] Iraji, F., Banan, L. 2010. The efficacy of nicotinamide gel 4% as an adjuvant therapy in the treatment of cutaneous erosions of pemphigus vulgaris. *Dermatol. Ther.* 23, 308-11.

[626] Vokurka, S., Skardova, J., Hruskova, R., Kabatova-Maxova, K., Svoboda, T., Bystricka, E., Steinerova, K., Koza, V. 2011. The effect of polyvinylpyrrolidone-sodium hyaluronate gel (Gelclair) on oral microbial colonization and pain control compared with other rinsing solutions in patients with oral mucositis after allogeneic stem cells transplantation. *Med. Sci. Monit.* 17, CR572-76.

[627] Rasero, L., Marsullo, M., Dal Molin, A. 2014. Assessing the effectiveness of Gelclair® in the prevention and therapy of stomatitis in patients undergoing hematopoietic stem-cell transplantation: a randomized trial. *Prof. Inferm.* 67, 15-20.

[628] Papas, A.S., Clark, R.E., Martuscelli, G., O´Loughlin, K.T., Johansen, E., Miller, K.B. 2003. A prospective, randomized trial for the prevention of mucositis in patients undergoing hematopoietic stem cell transplantation. *Bone Marrow Transplant.* 31, 705-12.

[629] Rao, N.G., Trotti, A., Kim, J., Schell, M.J., Zhao, X., Amdur, R.J., Brizel, D.M., Chambers, M.S., Caudell, J.J., Miyamoto, C., Rosenthal, D.I. Phase II multicenter trial of Caphosol for the reduction of mucositis in patients receiving radiation therapy for head and neck cancer. *Oral Oncol.* 50, 765-69.

[630] Svanberg, A., Ohrn, K., Birgegard, G. 2014. Caphosol® mouthwash gives no additional protection against oral mucositis compared to cryotherapy alone in stem cell transplantation. A pilot study. *Eur. J. Oncol. Nurs.* doi: 10. 1016/j.ejon.2014. 07. 01.

[631] Quinn, B. 2013. Efficacy of a supersaturated calcium phosphate oral rinse for the prevention and treatment of oral mucositis in patients receiving high-dose cancer therapy: a review of current data. *Eur. J. Cancer Care.* 22, 564-79.

INDEX